W9-COD-529

## SKIN MYTHS:

- Collagen creams firm skin
- More expensive products are better for your skin
- Wrinkled skin needs moisturizers
- Oily skin needs to be dried out
- Facial exercises tone up aging skin

## SKIN FACTS:

Fruit acids are the inexpensive, effective way to firm, moisturize and perfect your skin for a glowing, youthful complexion.

## FIND OUT HOW IN:

FRUIT ACIDS FOR FABULOUS SKIN

# FRUIT ACIDS

## FOR

# FABULOUS SKIN

## DEBORAH CHASE

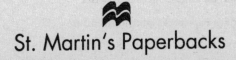

## St. Martin's Paperbacks

FRUIT ACIDS FOR FABULOUS SKIN

Copyright © 1996 by Deborah Chase.

Cover photograph courtesy Photonica.

ISBN: 0-312-95769-6

Printed in the United States of America

St. Martin's Paperbacks edition/April 1996

10  9  8  7  6  5  4  3  2  1

# Acknowledgments

This book could not have been written without the people who shared their time and expertise. I would like to thank especially Dr. Albert M. Lefkovits, of New York City whose intelligence and generosity of time provided the foundation for this book; Heather Jackson, the best editor a writer could have; Liz Hock whose enthusiasm and support helped to find a home for this project; Harvey Klinger, my agent whose energy and enthusiasm never failed to spur me on; Deborah and Peter Hughes for their emotional and editorial support; Nissa Simon who provided the access to research this book; Dr. Cherie Detrie of Philadelphia for her invaluable advice on the use of fruit acids on women of color; Dr. Helen Torok of Ohio for her information on fruit acid/ Retin-A combination therapy. Special thanks must go to Barbara Blauvelt for sharing her time and knowledge on the how's and why's of fruit acid peels.

# Author's Note

The products that appear in this book are intended to help the reader recognize the different forms and types of fruit acid beauty care products. I have personally tried all the face, skin, hair, nail and body products and have found them safe and effective. However, their appearance in the book does not constitute an endorsement, and neither I nor my publisher are responsible for any problems which may arise from their use.

The reader should keep in mind that the recipes at the end of each section contain active, fresh fruit acids and can be irritating to some people. Be careful to avoid the eye area, and remove quickly if a burning sensation develops. To prevent problems check with your dermatologist before adding homemade products to your skin- and hair-care routine. Because of the individuality of response, neither the author nor the publisher take responsibility for any problems that may arise from the use of these products.

# Table of Contents

# FRUIT ACIDS
# FOR
# FABULOUS SKIN

# Introduction

In the hall that runs between my bedroom and the living room I have hung a collection of cosmetic advertisements going back almost eighty years. Most of the illustrations feature society matrons and actresses solemnly and graciously proclaiming their loyalty to this soap or that cream, assuring the reader that these products meet their exacting standards. For decades, skin care and skin advertisements were fueled with equal measures of hope and glamour, and a dash of desperation. Then, seemingly overnight, care of the skin took a decidedly scientific bent, and the products and their ads became increasingly technical and medical. Instead of promises of softer skin or fewer lines and wrinkles, the ads were dotted with words like "cell renewal," "liposomes," "neosomes," and, my personal favorite, "trans-epidermal water loss."

The good news is that there are real advances behind the technobabble. The bad news is that these advances have led to increasingly complex scientific and medical terminologies that makes an ad in a beauty magazine sound more like a review sheet for an exam in medical school. I'm not sure if the cosmetics companies really don't understand how their products work or if they are just trying to make them sound better than they actually are. Whatever the reason, the resulting advertisements are often confusing and conflicting.

This incomprehensibility, coupled with past disappointments of other products, has created an understandable skepticism on the part of people reading of new beauty discoveries. This is unfortunate, because today we have a new approach to skin care that is widely available and is remarkably effective for a wide range of skin problems. It can even be produced in your own kitchen. This new discovery is fruit acids, or alpha hydroxy acids (AHAs), as they are more commonly known.

Use of fruit acids as part of a skin-care regimen is not completely new. Fruit acids are found naturally in a variety of foods including blackberries, tomatoes, sour milk or buttermilk, wine, and grapes. Women throughout the ages have recognized the potentials of these products. Cleopatra was reported to have bathed in sour milk to soften her sun-dried skin, a constant problem in hot, dry, desert climates. Women of the French court packed their faces with poultices of wine for the same results.

Many credit the start of the modern age of fruit acids to a paper published by Eugene Van Scott, M.D. The Philadelphia-based dermatologist was looking for new ways to treat a severe, actually disfiguring form of dry skin called ichthyosis. Traditional treatments had relied on a mixture of emollient creams and cell-dissolving agents, like salicylic acids and urea. Van Scott decided to look at other groups of compounds which might have a similar or better effect. In the early 1970s, he tested the effect of over sixty compounds and found that a group of fruit acids, even at relatively low concentrations, had exciting results.

## SOURCES OF FRUIT ACIDS

- Apples.............................Malic Acid
- Milk.................................Lactic Acid
- Sugar Cane...............Glycolic Acid
- Citrus Fruits..................Citric Acid
- Tomatoes.......................Lactic Acid
- Grapes, Wine............Tartaric Acid
- Blackberries...................Lactic Acid

The twelve fruit-acid compounds he tested were highly effective for relieving dryness and normalizing skin. What was particularly interesting was how quickly the fruit acids improved the patient's skin. Within two weeks of treatment, the dry, cracked skin fell away to reveal a healthy, normal skin surface. Van Scott was delighted with the results, but they only whetted his curiosity. While most women experience dry skin on some part of their body, icthyosis is a relatively rare condition. He reasoned that if fruit acids worked so well in treating disfiguring dry skin, they could easily relieve routine dryness. In the years that followed, Van Scott and other physicians have examined the effects of fruit acids on different types of skin problems. After two decades of study, we now have a good idea of how they work and under what circumstances they should be used.

Currently, there are hundreds of fruit acid–based products in pharmacies and department stores. Unfortunately, all products are not equal and one must select the right formulation in order to receive maximum benefits. Basic information about the skin—how it grows, how it gets into trouble, and what we can and cannot do—is needed to understand how best to use these products.

## Skin Care 101

The skin is built in layers, like a sandwich. The epidermis, the outermost level, is what we see when we look in the mirror. It is the part of the skin that blisters, flakes, burns, wrinkles, and breaks out. The dermis is the middle layer of the skin. This is the site of the collagen and elastin fibers which give the skin its strength and flexibility. Collagen fibers are colorless, wavy bands that are given their natural bounce by the way they weave together in the skin. Elastin fibers are small straight bands that can stretch out to twice their length and still spring back to their original size. As we become older both collagen and elastin tend to become stiff, tangled and frayed. Sadly the body is not inclined to repair damage to these vital fibers. Much of the sagging and wrinkling we see in older skin is the result of damaged and weakened collagen and elastin.

In addition to collagen and elastin, the dermis also contains blood vessels and oil glands. Below the dermis lie the fat and muscle that give the skin its bulk and structure.

The epidermis itself has four layers, and each layer has a different job to do. The bottom layer is the basal layer, where the new skin cells grow. As they get older, they move up through the different layers of the epidermis and undergo a variety of changes. One of the most important changes is the development and the increase of keratin protein. By the time new skin cells reach the top, they are composed entirely of dry, dead keratin. Although keratin is dead, it needs water to stay strong and flexible. If the water level drops too low, the keratin crumbles, the cells become loose and flaky, and the skin looks dry and rough.

The amount of water in the skin is dependent on the middle layer of the epidermis, called the stratum corneum. This region is thought to contain water-attracting compounds that we call NMFs, or natural moisturizing factors. As we grow older, the amount of NMFs in the skin decreases. This decline is believed to be one of the reasons that the skin becomes drier as the years go by.

When the cells reach the top layers of the epidermis, they are held together by oil, sweat, water, and cellular glue. This top layer is meant to be removed. Its removal actually stimulates the growth of cells in the lower growing layers of the skin. If it's not removed by proper washing, the skin begins to look dull and blotchy. This accumulated waste on the surface can also plug up pores and cause blackheads and blemishes.

## WHAT FRUIT ACIDS CAN DO

- Improve skin cell renewal
- Restore moisture to the skin
- Strengthen collagen and elastin fibers
- Improve skin texture and tone
- Reduce lines around the eyes
- Lighten brown spots of discolorations
- Soften dry, cracked soles of the feet
- Improve action of sunless tanners
- Reduce shaving irritation
- Improve results of waxing
- Remove nail cuticles without cutting
- Relieve dandruff
- Reverse signs of skin aging
- Reduce acne blemishes
- Brighten skin tone

In normal, healthy skin, thorough cleansing will remove just the right amount of the topmost layer to stimulate the lower layers to grow. In oily skin, the oil makes the skin cells stick together and become more difficult to remove. In dry skin, the cells are very loose, and too many cells are removed by washing. This may lead people to decrease the amount of cleansing, which then leads to a pileup of dead cells on the skin's surface. Problems with any of the layers of the skin can affect the way the skin is going to look and feel.

The single biggest threat to healthy skin is the sun, which damages the skin at almost every level and in almost unimaginable ways. There is an old adage that you can't tell the age of a woman by her bottom, because the age of the unexposed skin is years younger than that of the skin layer exposed to the environment. The sun's rays literally fray and crack collagen and elastin fibers. The heat of the sun damages blood vessels so they can no longer provide food and oxygen to the skin cells, which in turn slows down skin growth. The rays stimulate the production of melanin as well as abnormal cells which leads to blotchy, dark pigmentation and skin cancer. Finally, the destruction of the blood vessels decreases the healthy glow of the skin, producing a sallow, yellow skin tone.

## THE SCIENCE OF MODERN SKIN CARE

Most of the changes that we see in the skin either because of natural skin aging or sun damage are due to problems in the rate of skin growth. Skin care research has often focused on ways to regulate the way skin cells grow in order to resolve a wide range of beauty problems. Fruit acids are effective because they act to correct irregularities in skin growth.

The best way to understand the range of activity of fruit acids is to look at them as the aspirin of skin-care products. For example, if you take a couple aspirin, you can get rid of a simple headache or cool down a fever. Larger doses of aspirin are used to relieve the severe pain of rheumatoid arthritis. Recent studies have shown that one aspirin a day can decrease the risk of heart disease.

Similarly, different types of fruit acids at different concentrations can do different things to make the skin look better. Fruit acids remove the top, dead layer of skin cells that clog the surface. They achieve this naturally and gently, without stripping off oil or taking away water. This cleansing has two effects. The first is that it makes the skin look brighter and fresher, because the dulling layer is removed. Secondly, it stimulates the production of new, healthy cells, a process that we call cell renewal.

Cell renewal is a fascinating concept. Researchers credit the fact that men seem to age slower than women, not because they are physiologically superior, but because they shave every day. Removing the top layer of skin cells with a razor stimulates the lower layers to grow stronger and firmer tissue. Fruit acids have the same mechanical effect of stimulating skin-cell growth.

The second achievement of fruit acids is the stimulation of a natural moisturizing factor called glycosphingolipids, or GAGs. A single molecule of GAGs can hold a thousand times its weight in water—and it holds it in a very special way. With even the best moisturizers, water is held in the skin by placing a shield on the surface so water cannot evaporate. With GAGs, the water is held deep inside the cells, giving the skin a unique plumpness and softness that cannot be achieved with any other type of moisturizer.

More recently, researchers have discovered that fruit acids can actually stimulate the production of new collagen and elastin, those fibers that give the skin its strength and flexibility. We are all born with healthy, normal elastin and collagen. As we go through life, movement, sunlight, and usage permanently damage these essential fibers. The body has very little ability to replace them after adulthood. The collagen fibers that give our skin the ability to smile, laugh, talk, and eat just wear out. Fruit acids are thought to stimulate the production of new collagen and restructure and reorganize the elastin fibers, restoring a degree of strength and flexibility to the skin.

Fruit acids can be helpful for an extraordinary range of skin problems. They can be used to make dry skin softer, to reduce fine lines and wrinkles, to deal with acne-induced problems, to soften dry, cracked feet, and to lighten discolorations such as freckling and sun spots. Fruit acids are particularly fascinating in that they often act indirectly to improve the quality of skin. For example, added to sunless tanners, they don't make the skin darker, but they remove the top layer of skin cells. This allows for better penetration of the sunless tanner, so the resulting color is more even, deeper, and longer lasting.

## MYTH: EXPENSIVE SKIN-CARE PRODUCTS PRODUCE BETTER RESULTS

When it comes to fast cars, large rubies, and vintage champagne, price is an accurate guide to quality. With skin care it is a far less accurate predictor of performance. Whether or not a skin-care product will do its job depends on the ingredients, not price and packaging. Some products that cost forty dollars an ounce will do an excellent job; others that cost two dollars an ounce will perform equally well. In truth, there are effective and ineffective products at every price. For example, one of the most expensive fruit-acid lotions sold only in department stores contains less than two percent fruit acids. By contrast Freeman Sugar Cane and Guava Lotion with eight percent fruit acids weighs in at eighty cents an ounce. Avon Anew Intensive, an elegant ten-percent facial lotion, is a modest two dollars an ounce.

Before you throw down this book and run out to buy the first fruit acid you see, stop. Not all products deliver the same benefits. The outcome of using fruit acids depends on the best type for your individual skin need. The addition of fruit acids will also require major changes in your beauty routines. You cannot simply replace your current cleanser or moisturizer with a fruit-acid product. For example, if you have dry skin, your skin-care program may include saunas and face masks as well as day and night creams. All of these treatments are needed to remove dead skin cells, stimulate cell renewal, and rehydrate water-hungry skin. With fruit acids, most of these steps are unnecessary. The correct fruit-acid treatment product can accomplish these goals more effectively, in less time, and for less money.

In the next chapter we'll start to separate fact from fiction in the new world of fruit acids.

# Fruit Acids: Separating Fact from Fiction

After years of using beauty products that don't deliver, it is really hard to imagine just how attractive a well-designed fruit-acid product can make the skin look. The surface of the skin appears to retexturize, making it look firmer, softer, and fresher. The skin develops a luminous quality you may not have enjoyed since childhood.

The skin change from fruit acids can have a psychological effect that recalls an old French fable. A messy, old woman is given a beautiful white iris. She puts the iris in a vase and stands back to admire it. The iris is lovely, but she realizes the vase is dusty and cloudy. She takes the flower out and scrubs the vase down until it shines. She then puts the vase and the flower back on the table. She sees that the beauty of the vase brought out the fact that the table is dusty and cluttered. So she clears off all the papers and books and polishes the table until it glows. Then she puts the vase and the flower back. When she looks at her beautifully polished table and sparkling vase and fragrant white flower, she realizes the window behind it is dirty and the curtains look dusty and torn. So she takes them down to wash and polishes the window. Before long she has cleaned the whole house, inspired by the beauty of one flower.

I have seen this same effect happen to women after treatment with fruit acids. A woman saw her skin glow with such a fresh, luminous quality that she felt that it didn't go with her hair, which had become gray and scraggly. So she went out and got it freshly colored and cut. Then she recognized that her dowdy clothes didn't go with her new face and hair, so she dropped those ten pounds that made her look dumpy and brought home bright, new clothes—all because fruit acids made such a change in her skin.

## THE TRUTH ABOUT FRUIT ACIDS

Fruit acids are natural products. Although many companies now synthesize fruit acids, the natural effect of a natural product must be appreciated. There are five types of fruit acids that are frequently part of cosmetic formulas. Despite the term, not all of them come from fruit. Glycolic acids are found in sugar cane; lactic acid is found in sour milk, blackberries, and tomatoes; tartaric acid comes from grapes and wine; and citric acid derives from citrus fruits and pineapple. There is some evidence that lactic acid is particularly good for moisturizing your skin, and glycolic acid is the most effective at cell renewal. Both acids are often used interchangeably in a range of treatment products.

Because they both slow down skin aging and help acne problems there is a great deal of comparison between fruit acids and Retin-A. In truth, they perform very different actions on the skin. Retin-A works by taking off the top dead layers, dissolving them, and creating a very rapid growth process. This activity can cause extreme dryness, cracking, and irritation. Retin-A dilates blood vessels in the skin, significantly increasing circulation. This improved blood flow encourages growth of healthy young collagen, but produces a harsh, red skin tone. Finally, Retin-A makes the skin extremely sensitive to the sun. Even a short exposure can produce a damaging burn. If you use Retin-A you must stay out of the sun and use heavy sunscreens at all times. People who live in sunny climates like Arizona and Florida, who also endure the most serious sun damage, can find Retin-A difficult to use.

In contrast, fruit acids make the skin more luminous. They don't cause redness, but instead produce a natural, blushing glow. This is due not to increased circulation, but to the natural glow that is revealed when the dulling layer of old skin is removed. Fruit acids don't make your skin increasingly sensitive to the sun, so you can use them daily and still go out in the sunshine. Although we advise always using a sunscreen to prevent against sun damage, you needn't worry about getting a serious sunburn using fruit acids. Finally, you can't make Retin-A at home, but you can make many fruit-based tonics, cleansers, moisturizers, and masks in your own kitchen— with less time and money than it would take to make a quick snack.

Fruit-acid products are available from four sources: those you can make at home; commercial products that are available on drugstore or department store shelves; professional treatments and products available from physicians and cosmeticians; and product lines available by catalog and mail order.

There are over one hundred recipes in the upcoming chapters for fruit-acid treatments, including cleansers, lotions, toners, and masks. You can adjust the ingredients to meet your exact needs, adding a bit more soap or a touch less thickener. You will be able to create effective products that are not available in stores. For example, there are recipes for fruit-acid foot soaks, hair conditioners, and nail moisturizers that will work so well you will wonder why nobody thought of them before.

Prices for commercial fruit-acid products range from about a dollar to forty dollars per ounce, but the effectiveness is not based on price. Most doctors believe that a treatment product must contain at least five percent fruit acid in order to have an impact on the skin. Unfortunately for the consumer, price is unrelated to product strength. For example, one heavily-advertised fruit-acid gel is reported to contain less than two percent fruit acid and sells for forty dollars an ounce. By contrast, Pond's Age Defying Complex contains eight percent fruit acids and runs about five dollars an ounce.

Products available from both physicians and beauty specialists can contain between eight and twenty percent fruit acid. They also offer fruit-acid peels in their offices that use fifty to seventy percent fruit acid. The peeling solutions are put on for just a few minutes, then rinsed off. At the highest concentrations, many physicians believe that use of this treatment should be limited to doctors and not to lay cosmeticians, because there is the potential for injury if the technician lacks adequate skill and experience.

While there are numerous direct-mail companies that sell fruit-acid products, there are three companies which are widely respected and recommended by physicians: Murad (1-800-242-1103), M.D. Formulations (1-800-MD-FORMULA), and NeoStrata (1-800-628-9904). They each have an extensive line of products for a range of skin types and problems. With their products fairly priced, clearly labelled, and effective, they often offer products that are unavailable in retail drug and department stores. These mail-order companies readily share the concentration of their fruit-acid formulations, often listing the percentages right on the label or in the package insert—a policy that I wish some of the larger manufacturers would follow.

## PLAYING THE PERCENTAGES

Getting the results you want from fruit-acid treatments depends on using the right concentration in the appropriate base. Many cosmetic companies recognize the importance of this information to the consumer. They list the concentration of the product on the label or provide it through their consumer affairs departments. Others are uncomfortable discussing the concentrations of their fruit-acid products. This is a problem. Without this information there is no way of knowing if the product is too strong or too weak for your skin needs. Too strong, it can produce excessive peeling and irritation. Too weak and you will not receive the benefits that you should expect from fruit-acid treatment. While the lower strength fruit acids still remove a bit of dead skin, they certainly cannot produce the softening, clarifying, and toning benefits of the stronger products. This doesn't discourage a few companies from making such claims for their weaker products.

Some manufacturers claim that you can't judge the effectiveness of a fruit acid by its strength, and that its value lies in the other ingredients and techniques used in its production. The truth is that no matter how brilliantly it is conceived or what magnificent oils or waxes have been used, if a treatment product does not contain adequate fruit-acid levels— between five and ten percent—you are not going to see the improvements you should expect from a fruit acid. Low levels of fruit acids in soaps and cleansers are not as much of a problem. You want this product to thoroughly and gently clean the skin, and these mild fruit acids will do just that. Additionally, they are generally intended to be used with fruit-acid treatment products and thus are based on understanding the need to avoid irritating the skin.

More than a few cosmetic companies refuse to reveal their concentrations at all. While these may turn out to be excellent products, I am not comfortable with treatment lotions, gels, creams, or moisturizers that do not publish their strengths. If you do not know the strength, there is no way of knowing if the product is right for your skin needs. If there is a product that interests you, write or call the company and ask for the concentration or percentage of fruit acids. If they refuse to provide the strength of a formulation, look for one made by a company that is more sensitive to consumer needs.

Fruit acids are now found in over three hundred products used for nails, cuticle removers, sunless tanners, moisturizers, and cleansers. I can't say strongly enough that just because a product says it has a fruit acid, it doesn't mean that it's going to be helpful. I can't be at your side standing at drugstore counters and department stores as you look at the seemingly endless rows of bottles and jars. This book is designed to empower you to make the right decisions and choose the right products. It will help you sort out the different formulations to choose the ones that are best for you at the best possible price.

The treatment products listed in the book

contain at least five percent fruit acids. I have used all these products in the book and have found them safe and effective. They are not listed as an endorsement but as a guide to the type of product that you should look for for an individual problem. As I write this book, new fruit-acid products are introduced each month. Giving examples of the type of product I am describing can help you recognize and evaluate new products as they appear on the shelves.

Don't get frustrated and give up if products seem to become a blur. Start by writing down on a card your skin type, what kind of a product you want, and what strength you need. If you have dry skin are looking for a fruit-acid lotion with a sunscreen, gather all the products for your skin type. This eliminates all the ones that are designed for normal, oily, or acne-troubled skins. Now check the concentration of each item. If you are looking for a mild one, eliminate the products with more than six percent fruit acid. At this point you are probably down to two or three products, and you can't go wrong with any of your choices. You can now make your final selection on price, texture, or fragrance, confident that you will be getting the product that meets your needs.

# Typing Your Skin

The first step in choosing the right type of fruit acid is determining what shape your skin is in doing and what it needs. This is not as easy as it sounds. Many of us have misdiagnosed and mistreated our skins, due in no small measure to misinformation from cosmetic companies trying to sell us an ever greater number of products. For example, many women believe they have dry skin when they actually have normal or slightly oily skin. Conditioned to regard any sign of skin tightness as terminal dry skin, they pour on oils and moisturizers and stay away from soap. The result? Skin becomes dull and muddy, and breaks out. They wonder how their dry skin could be troubled with blemishes. Others never change their skin care routine from their teenage years. They continue using harsh soaps and cleansers to dry out what is now normal skin.

The first step in choosing a fruit acid is to take a skin analysis test. When choosing fruit acids it is helpful to divide skin into five types: normal, simple dry, complex dry, oily, and acne troubled. Notably absent in this list is the so-called combination skin. Actually all skins have areas that are drier or oilier than others. It is the general, overall skin condition that must be considered when choosing a skin-care program. If you moisturize drier areas of oily and normal skin, the oils and waxes will spread out and add unwanted lubrication to the already oil-rich areas of the skin. The result will be a complexion that appears dull, muddy, and prone to break out.

## IDENTIFYING SKIN TYPES

Look through all five skin profiles before starting to answer questions. To find a match, answer each query carefully. If you answer "Yes" more than half of the time, you have identified your own true skin type. If you answer yes to more than one type, you're going to need a second opinion. Ask your mother, sister, or close friend to answer the questions for you. Not infrequently, we lose objectivity about our skin and hair—and another pair of eyes can clear up any confusion.

## THE FIVE BASIC SKIN PROFILES

### Oily Skin Profile

1. Did you have a problem with acne during high school?
2. Does your hair tend to be oily?
3. Does your foundation tend to wear off within a few hours?
4. Do you wake up with an oily film on your nose, forehead, and chin?
5. Do you tan easily?

### Simple Dry Skin

1. Are you under thirty-five?
2. Is your hair dry?
3. Do your hands often feel tight and rough?
4. Does your skin feel tight after washing or showering?
5. Did your skin sail through adolescence with little or no acne problems?

## Complex Dry Skin Profile

1. Are you over thirty-five?
2. Do you have raised brown spots, large freckles, or reddish patches on your skin?
3. Have you developed lines around eyes and forehead?
4. Is your skin dull with a pale or yellowish tone?
5. Does your skin sag along the jawline?

## Normal Skin Profile

1. Do you have even skin color, free of red or dark patches?
2. Are you free of enlarged pores?
3. Did acne problems clear up after high school?
4. Does your hair stay fresh between shampoos?
5. Can you try new products without fear of irritation?

## Acne-Troubled Skin

1. Do new products tend to make your skin break out?
2. Did you have moderate to severe acne during high school?

3. Does your skin break out even if you are careful about your cleansing and diet?
4. Are you troubled by dandruff?
5. Did your parents have oily or acne-troubled skin?

## PROFILE CONFIRMATION

To confirm your diagnosis, you can follow a three-day skin-care elimination trial to let your true skin condition declare itself. You can start this on a Thursday night so that you don't have to display your emerging skin to the rest of the world.

1. Put away all products that you are currently using for your skin and hair. This includes cleansers, moisturizers, toners, eye creams, sunscreen, shampoos, conditioners, foundations, and lip gloss. You can still wear mascara and lipstick.
2. Clean your face at night and morning with a soapless cleanser like Cetaphil or clear glycerin soap.
3. Cleanse your hair with a simple, clear shampoo without additional conditioners. Rich conditioning formulas can drip down on the face to affect oiliness.
4. Avoid sun exposure. Your skin is not

protected, and you don't want to promote damage and aging.

5. After three days, examine your skin carefully in strong light. You should answer five key questions:

a. Is your skin oilier? (This means your skin is probably oily, since the mild soap you were using is really inadequate for cleansing oily skin.)

b. Does your skin look fresh and feel soft? (An indication that you have normal skin.)

c. Does your skin look dull and flaky? Are the fine lines more pronounced? (Signs that you have complex dry skin.)

d. Does your skin feel tight and irritated? (Clear signs of simple dry skin.)

e. Do you have fewer break outs? (This could mean that you have overused moisturizers on normal and oily skin.)

If your skin profile turns out to be different than the way you have been treating your skin, you will be very happily surprised by the way just simple changes in the treatment of your skin can make a difference. If you were right about your skin profile, you will be equally delighted by the improvements that fruit acids can provide over your current form of skin treatment

Fruit-acid products demand real changes in

your beauty regimens. For example, if you have oily skin, you are probably using strong soaps, cleansers, toners, or scrubbing grains. It might seem unsettling to give up all your trusted products for a simple cleanser and a single fruit-acid gel. If you have dry skin, fruit-acid skin care means putting away bath oils, thick night creams, and saunas for a single fruit-acid cream. It takes a leap of faith to alter radically time-honored beauty techniques, but you'll be glad you did when you see the results.

# Care of the Skin

## BEFORE YOU START

Before you crack an egg or squeeze a lemon, organize the tools and ingredients you will need to make fruit-acid beauty aids at home. Virtually everything you will need will be found in four locations—supermarkets, health food stores, drugstores, and housewares aisles.

## EQUIPMENT NEEDS

- small enamel pot—for melting oils and wax
- 8-oz. glass custard dish—these will be frequently used for melting creams and wax in the microwave
- small wire whisk—to whip ingredients together
- measuring spoons—to combine accurately ingredients

- funnel—to pour liquids into storage jars
- blender or food processor—to puree grapes, tomatoes, and apples
- hand juicer—to squeeze lemon juice
- glass bowls—for mixing ingredients
- measuring cups—to add correct amounts of liquids
- glass and plastic storage container in sizes that range from 4–16 ozs.
- labels and waterproof markers—to date and label products
- eyedropper—to be able to add small amounts of liquids

## INGREDIENTS:

Ingredient lists are divided into the stores where they can be found. No one will want all the items on the three lists. Check the ingredient list in each recipe section to identify the products that your skin or hair will need.

Health Food Stores: almond oil, aloe vera, apricot kernel oil, beeswax, castor oil, cocoa butter, coconut oil, lanolin, lecithin, sesame oil, vitamin C, wheatgerm oil.

Grocery Stores: alum, apples, blackberries, buttermilk, borax, Crisco, eggs, gelatin, grapes, honey, lemons, oatmeal, olive oil, sour cream, tomatoes, canned tomato juice, vinegar, yogurt.

Drug Stores: castile soap, boric acid powder, epsom salts, facial soap (liquid), glycerin, mineral oil, petroleum jelly, tincture of benzoin, witch hazel.

## Basic Rules of Kitchen Cosmetics

If you can make a cup of coffee or scramble up some eggs, you have the skill to prepare wonderful fruit-acid products at home. The basic rules of cooking apply, but with one extra consideration—you must be very careful to avoid contaminating the homemade beauty aids with unwanted bacteria. Take the ten rules of preparation seriously. Read them over several times before you start.

### The Ten Rules of Preparation

1. Wash down your tabletop with disinfectant spray and wipe dry with a disposable paper towel.
2. Wash hands carefully with antibacterial soap.
3. Run all bowls, jars and lids, whisks, measuring cups and spoons through a

dishwasher or boil them for five minutes in a large pot of water.

4. Wash all fruits and vegetables before combining them with other ingredients.
5. Store your preparations in clean jars with tight lids.
6. Label and date all products.
7. Store all preparations in a refrigerator.
8. When using a cream, don't use your fingers. Dip in a clean spoon and take out what you need.
9. Check the date on any product before you use it.
10. Discard within a week.

## NORMAL SKIN

If you ask women what type of skin they have, fewer than ten percent would check the box for normal. Maybe there's something that sounds a little boring or ordinary about having normal skin. That's too bad, because normal skin is strong, healthy, and slow to age. Normal skin is balanced. It produces enough oil to help the skin hold moisture in the cells. It is not prone to breakouts. It tans rather than burns. The pores are small and lines and wrinkles are minimal.

Many women under thirty-five have normal skin, but they don't know it. They abuse their skin, either drying it out with harsh soaps and toners or drowning it under oil-enriched cleansers. The aim to caring for normal skin is not to disrupt its own natural balance. You want to be able to cleanse, tone, and stimulate cell renewal without adding excess oil that will provoke breakouts—or drying the skin out so that it becomes flaky and rough.

It might seem odd to use a fruit acid for normal skin. After all, if the skin is normal, what help does it need? The truth is that fruit acids will enhance and reveal normal skin like no other product. It can produce a poreless, luminous quality to the skin that many women feel gives them better skin than they have ever had before. In addition, it can maintain the youth and freshness of the skin by encouraging a healthy water balance and stimulating the growth of collagen and elastin to keep the skin strong and flexible.

## FRUIT-ACID HOME CARE FOR NORMAL SKIN

The key words in any treatment program for normal skin are first "do no harm." The cleansing program should remove dirt, stale oil, and the top layer of dead skin cells without stripping skin of essential moisture. There are a wide range of cleansers for normal skin. Bar soap, oatmeal-based soap, and milky cleansers all work well as long as they are not too rich in oil or too high in alcohol. Some examples of good cleansers for normal skin include Milky Cleanser (Elizabeth Arden) and Neutrogena Facial Cleansing Formula. There are a few fruit-acid cleansers that can be nice additions to a treatment plan. The concentration of fruit acids, however, is usually low and some physicians believe that the cleansers are in contact with the skin too briefly to have an impact on skin health. Despite these reservations, they can fit nicely into a fruit-acid treatment program. Examples of commercial products for normal skin include Tangerine Dream (Rachel Perry) and Aqua Glycolic Facial Skin Cleanser (Herald Pharmacal). At home you can whip up blackberry summer cleanser, lemon honey soap, and buttermilk creamy cleanser.

In normal skin, the use of fruit acids can usually eliminate the need for toners. If your skin does not feel clean without one, you can use a mild commercial toner such as Dickinson's Witch Hazel. Make your own using white wine or vitamin C.

The best fruit-acid treatment for normal skin is a gel or lotion with a fruit-acid content of five to eight percent. Be sure to choose an oil-free formulation that will not clog the pores of normal skin. Examples of this type of product include Pond's Age Defying Complex and Kiss My Face Alpha Aloe.

## WARNING: DON'T BUY A FRUIT-ACID PRODUCT WITHOUT KNOWING ITS STRENGTH

Most experts agree that a fruit acid product must contain at least 5% acid to be an effective treatment product. While many commercial formulations meet this standard, others contain very little fruit acid or their manufacturers refuse to divulge the concentration of fruit acid. If the product contains inadequate amounts of fruit acid, you will not see the results you should expect from this type of treatment. If this information is not available, you will be unable to judge if the product is too weak or too strong for your needs. Look for the percentage of fruit acid on the label. If it's not there, call the manufacturer. Most will understand the importance of this information and be happy to provide it over the phone. If a cosmetic company refuses to supply the figures, go to one that will.

You still may need an oil-free moisturizer on top of the fruit-acid product. This moisturizer will provide the water for the natural moisturizing factors in the skin to grab on and hold. For additional benefit, you can look for a daytime moisturizer with a sunscreen such as

Neutrogena Moisture with SPF 15. At night, you don't need sunscreen, but can still benefit from an oil-free lotion such as Complex 15 (Key Pharmaceutical).

Facial masks fortified with fruit acids will round out your home treatment plans. Commercial masks for normal skin include Sally Hansen Purifying Facial Mask and Naturistics Alpha Natural Skin Renewal.

## PROGRAM OF CARE FOR NORMAL SKIN

There are two basic styles of cleaning the skin. Program A works well if you tend not to wear foundation or cream blush, while Program B works particularly well if you wear foundation and/or face powder. You will note that both programs call for a "time-out" between washing the face and application of the fruit-acid gel or lotion. This rest period prevents burning or irritation from the fruit acids. Don't skip it.

### Nighttime Program A

1. Remove eye makeup with nonoily eye area cleanser.
2. Moisten a bar of facial soap with water and work up a lather with your hands.

3. Massage gently into skin, then rinse off with handfuls of warm water.
4. Finish with a final rinse of three handfuls of cool—not cold—water.
5. Dry gently and wait 10 minutes.
6. Apply fruit-acid gel or lotion to face and neck, excluding eye area. If the face feels irritated or stings, apply a simple, light, oil-free moisturizer.

## Nighttime Program B

1. Remove eye makeup with nonoily cleanser.
2. Apply a rinseable cleanser to the skin according to directions. Rinse off thoroughly, ending with four handfuls of cool—not cold—water.
3. Pat face dry. Wait 10 minutes.
4. Apply facial fruit-acid lotion or gel to the rest of the neck and face. If skin feels irritated, apply oil-free moisturizer.

## Daytime

1. Cleanse skin with rinseable cleanser or mild soap. Do not use deodorant soap on your face (if that's what you use in the shower).

2. Dry the face gently.
3. Wait 10 minutes, then apply fruit-acid facial lotion.
4. If skin feels irritated, apply oil-free moisturizer with sunscreen.
5. Even out skin tones and add further protection with sunscreen-enriched foundation.

## Weekly Facial

1. Wet face and work up lather with rinseable cleanser for normal skin.
2. Apply fruit acid–based mask. Leave on according to directions.
3. Rinse off mask.
4. Dry gently. Wait 15 minutes.
5. Apply fruit acid–enriched lotion or gel.

## PROFESSIONAL CARE

Office-based treatments from physicians or cosmeticians offer a series of fruit-acid peels. The peels "jump start" skin improvement removing the top dead layer that dulls and ages a complexion.

For most skin types, office peels correct problems such as clogged pores and discolorations. In the case of normal skin the office peel prevents rather than corrects problems. At first, the highly concentrated gel is used for as little as one minute, until the skin becomes adapted to the stronger concentrations. Over a course of several weeks, the length of time is gradually increased up to nine to ten minutes, depending on skin type. This treatment speeds up the results that are achieved with the lower concentration of home-use products. After a regular course of treatment that usually lasts from four to six weeks, the improvements can be maintained by regular home use of standard strength fruit-acid products. Many experts recommend booster skin-peel treatments three to four times a year.

## FRUIT-ACID RECIPES FOR NORMAL SKIN

Be sure to read the section on "before you start." Check that you have all the ingredients you need and all the equipment is clean and ready to use. You can mix and match commercial and homemade products; for example, use a cleanser from a drugstore and finish up with your own lemon toner.

## Normal Skin Ingredients List:

Almond oil, aloe vera gel, apple juice, blackberries, egg white, gelatin, glycerin, honey, liquid facial soap, lemon juice, lecithin, mint (fresh), olive oil, parsley, red grapes, rosemary (dried), sesame oil, tomato juice, vitamin C tablets, wheat germ oil, white wine, wheat germ, yogurt (low fat).

### BLACKBERRY SUMMER CLEANSER

6 ripe blackberries, crushed
2 teaspoons almond oil
3 teaspoons witch hazel solution

- Whip all ingredients together in a blender or miniprocessor.
- Spread onto the face and massage into skin lightly.
- Rinse off with warm water, followed by a few handfuls of cool water.

### LEMON HONEY SOAP

1 tablespoon liquid facial soap
2 tablespoons honey
2 tablespoons lemon juice

- Stir, but do not beat together all ingredients.
- Massage into skin.
- Rinse thoroughly with lukewarm water.

## MILKY CLEANSER

2 tablespoons aloe vera gel
1 tablespoon buttermilk or plain low-fat yogurt

- Mix ingredients together.
- Massage into skin.
- Rinse off with cool water.

## TUSCAN NIGHT CREAM

$\frac{1}{2}$ oz. beeswax
2 tablespoons light olive oil
4 tablespoons tomato juice
$\frac{1}{2}$ teaspoon lecithin

- Melt all ingredients together over low heat.
- Remove from heat and place over a bowl of cool water.
- Beat vigorously until mixture is creamy.
- Transfer cream to small plastic container with lid.
- To use, massage about a teaspoon into skin after cleansing face.

### HERBAL BUTTERMILK LOTION

3 tablespoons chopped parsley
1 tablespoon chopped fresh mint
1 cup buttermilk

- Steep herbs in buttermilk for 2 hours (keep in refrigerator).
- Strain, discarding herbs.
- Dab buttermilk onto clean face with cotton ball.
- After 10 minutes, apply foundation or makeup if you wish.

### APPLE CREAM

1 tablespoon apple juice
1 teaspoon glycerin
1 tablespoon sweet almond oil

- Stir and blend all ingredients over low heat.
- Transfer to a small plastic container.
- To use, massage a few drops onto freshly-washed skin before going to sleep.

### VITAMIN FRESHENER

1 cup boiling water
1 vitamin C tablet
1 teaspoon liquid glycerin

- Dissolve tablet in boiling water.
- Refrigerate until cold; transfer to a clean glass bottle.
- Apply to clean skin with a cotton ball.
- Store remainder in refrigerator.

## ROSEMARY TONER

2 cups white wine
1 tablespoon dried rosemary leaves

- Boil wine and rosemary together for 10 minutes.
- Cool for 30 minutes, then strain.
- Transfer steeped wine to a dark glass container and store in the refrigerator.
- To use, saturate a cotton ball with toner and smooth on the face.

## TOMATO MASK

2 tablespoons tomato juice
1 tablespoon wheat germ

- Mix ingredients together.
- Apply to face.
- Allow mask to remain for 20 minutes.
- Rinse off with cool water.

## APPLE GEL MASK

1 packet gelatin
$\frac{1}{2}$ cup apple juice

- Combine gelatin and juice.
- Heat for 45 seconds in a microwave, or 3–5 minutes on a stove.
- Cool until almost set.
- Spread on face.
- Allow to remain for 20 minutes.
- Rinse off with handfuls of warm water, followed by splashes of cool water.

## GRAPE FACE MASK

$\frac{1}{2}$ cup red grapes, ground
1 teaspoon lemon juice
1 teaspoon sesame oil
1 teaspoon wheat germ oil
1 egg white, lightly beaten

- Mix all ingredients together.
- Apply to face with a cotton ball.
- Allow to remain for 20 minutes.
- Rinse off with lukewarm water, followed by generous handfuls of cool water.

# FRUIT-ACID PRODUCTS FOR NORMAL SKIN

CLEANSERS:
Murad AHA Exfoliant Cleanser
Alpha Hydrox Foaming Cleanser
Alpha-Natural Facial Soap

TREATMENT PRODUCTS:
Avon Intensive for Face (10%)
Elizabeth Arden Alpha Ceramide (7.5%)
Alpha Hydrox Face Lotion (6%)
NeoStrata AHA Skin Smoothing Cream
Formula 405 AHA Facial Day Cream (6%)

TONERS:
Andrea Sensations Clarifying Toner

MASKS:
Diane Young Fruit Acid Concentrate
Sally Hansen Skin Recovery Purifying Mask
Naturistics Alpha Natural Skin Renewal

## OILY SKIN

Oily skin is something of a mixed blessing. On the plus side, it is slow to develop discolorations, fine lines, and wrinkles. Oily skin usually tans beautifully, rather than just burning and turning red. It has less of a tendency to freckle. On the downside, oily skin can look dull and muddy. It is prone to breakouts even when a woman is well past her teens, and large pores can develop that make the skin look coarse and rough.

Oil glands in the skin have a hair-trigger response and can be stimulated by factors both inside and outside the body. Hormones, foods that are high in fat, as well as hot, humid weather can provoke oil glands to work overtime.

The traditional approach to caring for oily skin has been to use cleansers and toners that strip the skin of all available oil, and scrubbing grains to remove some of the cellular debris that builds up on the surface. Results are not always that wonderful. Frequently, this type of aggressive cleaning leaves the skin dry and irritated. Some women maintain that when they remove the oil from the skin, it actually seems to stimulate the oil glands to produce even more oil a few hours later.

Fruit acids don't dissolve the oil, nor do they stop the skin from producing oil. Rather, they work on removing the top dead layer of skin, which is a combination of stale oil and dead, dry cells. This removal takes away the excessive oils without stripping the body of its natural moisture. Moreover, the removal of this layer stimulates the lower skin levels to produce a healthy, normal level of skin growth. Fruit acids may help diminish obvious pores because this top dead layer often becomes caught in the follicle, stretching the opening. By keeping the pores free of unwanted material, the pores can shrink in size.

The use of fruit acids for oily skin will refine and brighten the complexion, making it look soft, less oily, and smoother. One final bonus is the effect on water balance. All skin needs moisture—whether it be normal, dry, or oily. In the traditional treatment of oily skin we remove this moisture when we remove the oil. Fruit acids stimulate the skin to produce natural moisturizing factors that help the skin hold its own water. In fact, each molecule of the natural moisturizing factor stimulated by a fruit acid holds a thousand times its weight in water. The result is a natural plump texture without excessive oiliness.

---

**WARNING: DO NOT CLEANSE YOUR
FACE WITH STRONG SCRUBBING GRAINS
OR ABRASIVE SPONGES IF YOU ARE
USING FRUIT ACIDS**

Before we had fruit acids, scrubbing grains and
sponges were essential for thoroughly cleaning
the face as well as stimulating cell renewal. Today these needs are met with fruit-acid peels
and treatment products. Abrasive cleansers are
no longer necessary, and would be extremely
irritating for most fruit acid–treated skin.

---

Fruit acids do not replace a good program of
cleansing, toning, and sun protection. Rather,
they are a valuable addition to a balanced
treatment program. When you choose fruit
acids for oily skin, it is essential that you
choose oil-free products. Be very careful, because the majority of fruit-acid beauty products on the market are designed for normal or
dry skin. These formulations contain generous
amounts of waxes and oils, the last ingredients
oily skin needs. Despite the presence of fruit
acids in these products, the result will not be
good for oily skin. Examples of acceptable
fruit acid treatments for oily skin include:
Pond's Age Defying Complex, NeoStrata
AHA Solution for Oily Skin, and Kiss My Face
Alpha Aloe.

## FRUIT-ACID HOME CARE FOR OILY SKIN

When using a fruit-acid product on oily skin, you will probably need to change the way you wash your face. It's a safe bet that you are in the habit of using a combination of scrubbing grains, strong soaps, alcohol-based toners, and drying clay masks. Chances are most of these excellent products are going to be too harsh and drying when using fruit-acid gels. Happily, you won't need them. All their benefits—including degreasing, dead-skin removal, and cell renewal—will be accomplished by a fruit-acid regimen. Don't go overboard and switch to products that are rich in oils and waxlike, heavy moisturizers or creamy cleaners.

The solution? Change your skin-care program one step at a time. If you are using a liquid cleanser for oily skin try one for normal skin, such as Neutrogena Foaming Facial Cleanser. If you use a drying soap, try switching to a similar product designed for normal skin. There are only a few commercial fruit cleansers. Most are quite mild, and can be used by those with all but the driest skin. One added benefit—they are designed to be used with other fruit-acid products, so they are formulated to be non-irritating. Two excellent examples for oily skin are Freeman Sugar Cane and Guava Soap and Rachel Perry's Tangerine Dream.

---

## MYTH: OILY SKIN NEEDS A MOISTURIZER

Skin needs moisture to keep it from becoming dry, rough, and flaky. It loses this moisture through evaporation at the skin's surface. This water loss occurs primarily when the skin lacks a natural protective coat of oil . . . something that oily skin hardly lacks. One of the leading causes of acne in adult women is the needless use of creamy moisturizers and lotions on their faces.

If oily skin is coated with moisturizers and lotions, the skin will rebel with blackheads and blemishes. It's an all-too-common problem. In fact, many dermatologists believe that the needless use of moisturizers is one of the leading causes of acne in adults.

---

Fruit acid–based masks can be used on a weekly basis to absorb excess oil, as well as to deliver a steady, intense dose of fruit acids to the skin. Currently, most of the commercial masks are designed for oily and normal skin. This product group includes Freeman Sugar Cane and Guava Mask; Alpha Hydrox Peel-

Off Mask, and Sally Hansen Skin Recovery Purifying Facial Mask.

Don't forget to use a sunscreen as part of your skin-care treatment. Although oily skin is slower to age, nobody needs to absorb unnecessary light rays. Just by sitting in a sunny window or walking down a sunny street—particularly if you live in a high-sun region like Arizona, California, or Texas—your skin will absorb aging rays of sunlight. You can choose an oil-free sunscreen such as PreSun Active Clear Gel 15 (Westwood) or wear a foundation fortified with a sunscreen. One of the most interesting new products uses mechanical rather than chemical sunscreens. Total Coverage by Estée Lauder adds a microfine form of zinc oxide protection that provides a cosmetically beautiful foundationlike finish to the skin, while it offers extremely gentle yet very effective protection from the sun.

## FRUIT-ACID PROGRAM OF HOME CARE FOR OILY SKIN

There are several ways to take care of oily skin. It can be helpful to experiment with the different combinations to get the right balance of cleansing and cell renewal.

For example, if you have slightly oily skin

and usually clean your face with a clear glycerine soap for oily skin and follow up with a strong alcohol-based freshener, try instead a glycerine soap for normal skin and a fruit acid–rich toner. If your skin still doesn't feel clean, go back to your original cleanser with the fruit-acid toner. If your skin feels too tight and dry, keep using the soap for normal skin and eliminate the toner.

Keep in mind, changes in climate can have a major impact on oily skin. In hot, humid weather—which provokes the oil glands—you might need stronger cleansers and toners. In dry, cold weather, you may need to step down to milder cleansing and eliminate a toner entirely.

## Nighttime Program A

1. Carefully remove eye makeup with nonoily eye-area cleanser.
2. Work up lather from bar soap.
3. Massage lather into face; cleanse thoroughly. If lather starts to dry up, add more water.
4. Rinse off thoroughly, first with warm, then with a few handfuls of cool water.
5. Gently, but thoroughly dry the face with a clean, soft towel. Wait 15 minutes.

6. Apply toner with cotton ball. Wait another 2 minutes.
7. Apply oil-free fruit-acid lotion or gel.

## Nighttime Program B

1. Carefully remove eye makeup with nonoily eye-area cleanser.
2. Squeeze about three-quarters of a teaspoon of liquid cleanser into palm of the hand. Add warm water to work up a lather.
3. Massage into skin.
4. Rinse off thoroughly; first with warm water, finishing with cold.
5. Dry gently.
6. Wait 15 minutes.
7. Apply oil-free fruit-acid lotion.

## Daytime Program A

1. Cleanse with bar soap or rinseable cleanser.
2. Dry face with soft towel.
3. Apply toner with cotton ball.
4. Wait 15 minutes.
5. Dab on fruit-acid lotion or gel.
6. Apply sunscreen or sunscreen-enhanced foundation.

## Daytime Program B

1. Cleanse with bar soap or rinseable cleanser.
2. Dry face.
3. Wait 15 minutes.
4. Apply fruit-acid lotion.
5. Wait 5 minutes.
6. Apply sunscreen and/or foundation with sunscreen.

## Weekly At-Home Facials

Traditional facials include steaming and scrubbing grains. These steps are designed to remove the top dead layer of skin to promote cell renewal. With fruit acids, these steps are unnecessary and can cause unwanted irritation. Instead, follow the treatment plan below.

1. Wash face gently with cleanser of your choice.
2. Rinse with handfuls of warm water.
3. Apply fruit-acid mask.
4. Allow mask to remain up to 20 minutes.
5. Rinse off with cool water.
6. Gently pat face dry.
7. Smooth on fruit-acid gel or oil-free lotion.
8. Top with oil-free moisturizer.

## PROFESSIONAL FRUIT-ACID CARE FOR OILY SKIN

Oily skin can benefit from a series of office peels. Excessive oil glues the top layer of dead cells together on the skin surface, making the skin look dull and muddy. This layer not only looks bad, it is bad for skin growth, slowing down cell renewal. The result? The skin looks old and tired.

This thick, coarse skin responds beautifully to a series of seventy percent glycolic acid peels. Dermatologists dab a cotton ball soaked with a seventy percent–fruit acid solution on the forehead, nose, cheeks, and chin. The eye area is carefully avoided. At first, the solution remains on the skin for just three minutes, and then is rinsed off with cool water. Even after just one treatment you will see a clearing and brightening of the skin. The following day you might see a bit of peeling on the upper lip and cheeks.

Over the next few weeks, the length of treatment is gradually increased to nine minutes. Between visits, the dermatologist will often provide an eight-to-twelve-percent-fruit-acid cream to continue the improvements at home. If you are troubled by periodic breakouts or large pores on cheeks and chin, peels can be essential for retexturing and clarifying the skin's appearance.

## FRUIT-ACID RECIPES FOR OILY SKIN

In many ways oily skin is strong and resilient. It is slow to age, tans rather than burns, and can take advantage of strong fruit-acid formulations. Its vulnerability? Oil-rich formulations. We cannot use oils and cream as a base for the fruit-acid products you make at home. For this reason we cannot make a non-sticky oil-free fruit-acid gel or lotion. You can use commercial treatment gels in a daily regimen combined with toners and masks that you mix yourself.

### Oily Skin Ingredient Shopping List:

Aloe vera, borax, buttermilk, egg white, gelatin, honey, rice flour, soapless cleansers, thyme (dried), rosemary (dried), tomato juice, vodka, yogurt (fat free).

#### MILKY CLEANSER

¼ cup aloe vera
2 tablespoons fat-free yogurt
¼ tablespoon borax

- Mix ingredients together.
- Massage into skin.
- Rinse off with cool water.

## HONEY-TOMATO CLEANSER

1 tablespoon soapless cleanser
1 tablespoon honey
2 tablespoons tomato juice
¼ teaspoon borax

- Stir ingredients together.
- Transfer to small plastic container.
- Scoop out 1 tablespoon and massage into skin.
- Rinse off with warm, then cool water.
- Store remaining cleanser in refrigerator. After 1 week discard contents and save the jar.

## NAPA VALLEY NIGHT CARE

1 egg white
1 tablespoon white wine

- Whip ingredients together to a froth.
- Spread on the skin.
- Allow mask to remain on all night.
- Rinse off with lukewarm water.

## HERBAL TONER

1 teaspoon rosemary
1 teaspoon thyme
1 bay leaf
1 cup white wine

- Boil herbs with white wine for 10 minutes.
- Steep for 1 hour.
- Strain off herbs and discard them.
- Transfer toner to clean glass jar and store in refrigerator (up to one week).
- To use, saturate cotton ball in toner.
- Dab onto freshly-washed skin.

### BLOODY MARY TONER

1 tablespoon vodka
3 tablespoons water
1 tablespoon tomato juice
¼ teaspoon borax

- Mix all ingredients together.
- Apply with cotton ball.
- Transfer toner to clean glass bottle.
- Store in refrigerator.

### TUSCAN GEL MASK

1 packet gelatin
½ cup tomato juice

- Combine gelatin and tomato juice.
- Heat 45 seconds in the microwave or 2–3 minutes on stove.
- Stir until gelatin dissolves.
- Cool until almost set.
- Spread on face.

- Allow to dry for 30 minutes.
- Rinse off with warm, then cool water.

### DAIRYMAID MILK MASK

1 tablespoon buttermilk
1 egg white, beaten
1 teaspoon honey
1 teaspoon rice flour

- Blend all ingredients together.
- Smooth mixture on the face.
- Allow to dry for 30 minutes.
- Rinse off with cool water.

# FRUIT-ACID PRODUCTS FOR OILY SKIN

**CLEANSERS:**
Freeman Sugar Cane and Guava Soap
Aqua Glycolic Facial Skin Cleanser
Freeman Beautiful Skin Pineapple and Papaya
Foaming Enzyme Facial Wash

**TREATMENT PRODUCTS:**
Avon Anew
Murad Advanced Oily-Prone Skin
Kiss My Face Alpha Aloe
Alpha Hydrox Oil-Free Gel

**TONERS:**
Aqua Glycolic Astringent
Andrea Sensations Clarifying Toner Gel

**MASKS:**
Freeman Sugar Cane and Guava Mask
Alpha Hydrox Peel-Off Mask
Diane Young Fruit Acid Concentrate

## SIMPLE DRY SKIN

To judge by the number of products sold for dry skin, you might think it was a national health problem. Part of the concern about dry skin comes from the belief that dry skin causes aging. Not true. Dry skin is not a cause but a signal that the skin is more vulnerable to lines, wrinkles, and brown spots. Despite the attention paid to dry skin, few women realize there are actually two distinct types, simple dry skin and complex dry skin. They are caused by different factors and need different types of care. Simple dry skin is usually found in women under thirty-five. This skin was clear through adolescence without oily skin and breakouts, but began showing fine lines around the eyes and lips years earlier than women with oily skin. Simple dry skin often burns easily, and also can be sensitive to alcohol or alcohol based products. By contrast, complex dry skin occurs primarily in women over thirty-five.

The lack of natural oils is the driving force behind simple dry skin. Without adequate oil, the skin is unable to hold on to essential moisture. The result: The skin becomes dry, flaky, and dull.

Why we lack oil varies from woman to woman. In some cases, there may be fewer oil glands. In others, they may be ample in number but are lazy, producing inadequate amounts of oil. Production, however, is not the whole story. Skin health is heavily dependent on a group of chemicals that we call natural moisturizing factors. These naturally occurring substances, nicknamed NMFs, help the skin attract and hold on to moisture. The bad news is people with youthful, dry skin have lower levels of natural moisturizing factors. The good news is that fruit acids stimulate the production of some of the most powerful NMFs.

## MYTH: DRY SKIN CAUSES WRINKLES

We have been repeatedly told that dry skin causes lines and wrinkles—and that if we use enough creams and lotions, these problems can be avoided. Not true. The problems of skin aging—including wrinkling, sagging, dryness, pallor, and brown spots—are due to natural changes as the years go by. Dry skin develops as we stop producing both oil and natural moisturizing factors, while wrinkles are due to the breakdown of elastin and collagen fibers. Even if you drown your skin in moisturizers, you won't alter the aging process. What will help is protection from the sun. It is estimated that up to seventy percent of skin aging is actually sun damage. If you consistently use an effective sunscreen, you can prevent or at least limit the appearance of lines, wrinkles, and changes in skin color and texture.

The thrust of dry skin care has been to use mild cleansers that leave some oil and moisture in the skin, and moisturizers to put a shield on the surface to slow down water evaporation. Anyone who has used traditional moisturizers knows that the effect can be very short-lived. Cell renewal is also a problem for simple dry skin. The dull, flaky texture would benefit from scrubbing grains and abrasive sponges, but is too delicate to tolerate the treatment. Fruit acids are valuable for dry skins in two ways. They start by removing the top dead layer of dulling skin cells without stripping oil and water. In the skin, they stimulate the production of a type of NMF called glycosphingolipids or GAGs for short. One molecule of a GAG can hold a thousand times its weight in water. This is important water because it is deep in the skin, and it creates deep and long-lasting moisture.

With fruit acids, the body is stimulated to produce its own moisturizing factors, encouraging hydration long after the physical moisturizer has evaporated. Fruit acids feed water to each and every cell. This doesn't just make the surface smooth, but it holds water throughout the skin, producing a luminous, smooth quality.

It is hard to overstate the benefits of fruit acids for simple dry skin. The earlier you start using fruit acids, the more it will slow aging. Fruit acids are a gentle and effective way to improve cell renewal. Simple dry skin cannot tolerate the traditional cell-renewal methods that use scrubbing grains and abrasive sponges. As a result, gentle cleansing methods could not remove the top layer of dead cells, slowing skin growth. Fruit acids carefully dissolve the glue that holds the layer together, spurring a healthy youthful rate of skin cell development.

There are more fruit-acid products for dry skin than for any skin type. When using fruit acids, simple dry skin needs particularly gentle cleansing. The best choice would be a creamy, rinseable cleanser like Pond's Foaming Cleanser and Alpha Hydrox Foaming Cleanser, both of which contain small amounts of fruit acids. If your skin is particularly dry or easily irritated, you can use a similar cleanser like Neutrogena Cleansing Wash that does not contain fruit acids. Toners, even mild ones, are unnecessary and irritating for fruit acid–treated simple dry skin.

Fruit-acid masks can be a good source of moisture, but the commercial ones so far are too harsh for dry skin. Fortunately, you can easily make effective products in your home with the recipes that follow at the end of this chapter.

The key fruit-acid treatment is the lotion or cream that you choose to apply in the morning and before going to bed. You should look for a moisturizing product that contains between six and ten percent fruit acids. There is a wide selection of products to choose from that usually range from two dollars to forty dollars per ounce. Several well-designed products for simple dry skin include Avon Anew Intensive

for the Face, Neutrogena Healthy Skin, and
Murad Night Cream.

---

## MYTH: COLLAGEN CREAMS FIRM THE SKIN

Collagen fibers give the skin its strength and
flexibility. The ground-up animal collagen fibers that are incorporated into night creams
and moisturizers cannot restore your damaged
collagen. Sunlight and use has hardened and
splintered the ordered structure that gives
these fibers their natural bounce. Collagen ad-
ditives can, at best, act like any other routine
moisturizer, and slow down evaporation of water from the skin.

---

At night, plan on using a gentle moisturizer
over the fruit-acid cream. Although fruit acids
are the best moisturizing agents we have, most
doctors advise adding a moisturizer to a daily
skin-care program. This is not to hydrate the
skin but to reduce the chance of irritation and
inflammation. Simple dry skin is often thin
and fine, and particularly vulnerable to the
burning sensation that can accompany fruit-
acid products. For morning care look for a
moisturizer that also provides sun protection.

Examples of this include Eucercin Dry Skin Therapy SPF 25 and Nivea Visage SPF 8.

## FRUIT-ACID HOME CARE OF SIMPLE DRY SKIN

The regimen for simple dry skin is, well, simple. Don't worry, it works. Be sure to follow waiting periods between cleansing and application of a fruit-acid cream or lotion. Washing the skin even with gentle products opens the pores, leaving the skin bare and vulnerable to irritation. At this point, fruit acids can produce a burning, stinging sensation. Waiting from five to fifteen minutes allows the skin to stabilize and close the pores. The waiting time allows you to use a strong, highly effective fruit-acid formula without discomfort.

### Nighttime

1. Gently remove eye makeup with nonoily eye-makeup remover.
2. Squeeze a quarter-sized drop of rinseable cleanser into palm of hand. Add a few drops of water and massage into the skin. Never put the cleanser directly on your face as it can be irritating.

3. Rinse with 4 handfuls of warm water, followed by 3 handfuls of cool water.
4. Dry skin gently.
5. Wait 15 minutes.
6. Pat on fruit-acid cream.
7. Top with creamy moisturizer.

## Daytime

1. Cleanse face with rinseable cream or lotion.
2. Pat face dry gently.
3. Wait 15 minutes.
4. Apply a fruit-acid cream.
5. When fruit acid is absorbed, top with moisturizer that contains a sunscreen.

## Weekly Facial

1. Wash face with creamy rinseable cleanser.
2. Apply a moisturizing fruit-acid mask. Use the recipe at the end of this chapter.
3. Allow mask to harden and set for 20 minutes.
4. Gently rinse off with cool water.
5. Pat dry, wait 15 minutes.
6. Apply fruit-acid cream.
7. When cream is absorbed, apply moisturizer.

## FRUIT-ACID RECIPES FOR SIMPLE DRY SKIN

You can make just about every fruit-acid product you need in your own kitchen. In fact the only way to get fruit-acid toners and masks for your skin needs is to formulate them yourself. Be creative and combine commercial and homemade products in your skin regimen. For example you can start off with Napa Valley Cleansing Cream, and follow up with Oil of Olay Replenishing Cream. Have fun!

## <u>Ingredient Shopping List:</u>

Almond oil, apple juice, beeswax, borax, buttermilk, chervil (dried), egg, glycerin, honey, lanolin, lemons, mineral oil, olive oil, powdered skim milk, rosemary (dried), rose water, thyme (dried), vodka, Vaseline, white wine, witch hazel, yogurt, whole milk.

### LIQUID CLEANSER

1 tablespoon lanolin
2 tablespoons glycerin
1 tablespoon mineral oil
2 tablespoons apple juice
$\frac{1}{2}$ teaspoon borax

- Mix ingredients together.
- Transfer to clean jar with a lid.
- Store in refrigerator for up to 3 days.
- To use, massage 1 teaspoon into skin, rinse off with warm water.

## NAPA VALLEY CLEANSING CREAM

4 teaspoons beeswax
2 tablespoons white grape juice
½ teaspoon borax
1 tablespoon mineral oil

- Melt beeswax over low heat.
- Warm mineral oil and beat into wax mixture.
- Dissolve borax in warm grape juice.
- Combine all ingredients.
- Beat slowly until cool and creamy.
- Store in a covered jar in the refrigerator.
- To use, remove a nickel-sized dab in the hand and massage into the skin.
- Rinse off with warm water.

## DIXIE NIGHT CREAM

1 teaspoon almond oil
1 teaspoon glycerin
1 baked sweet potato
2 tablespoons whole-milk yogurt

- Combine almond oil and glycerin.
- Add sweet potato to glycerin mixture.
- Blend in yogurt.
- Spread on face.
- Store extra cream in a clean jar in refrigerator.
- Use within 2 days.

### LEMON DAY CREAM

1 tablespoon lanolin
1 tablespoon mineral oil
1 tablespoon Vaseline
1 tablespoon lemon juice
1 tablespoon vodka
½ teaspoon borax

- Melt lanolin and Vaseline.
- Warm mineral oil and beat into lanolin mixture.
- Add lemon juice and remaining ingredients.
- Beat until cool and creamy.
- Transfer to clean jar with a lid. Store in refrigerator for up to 1 week.

### HERBAL TONER

1 teaspoon dried chervil
1 teaspoon dried rosemary
1 teaspoon dried thyme

1 cup white wine
1 teaspoon glycerin

- Boil herbs in wine for 10 minutes.
- Steep for 30 minutes, then strain.
- Store toner in refrigerator.
- To use, dampen cotton ball with toner and apply to face.

### APPLE FRESHENER

2 tablespoons apple juice
2 tablespoons witch hazel
2 tablespoons rose water
1 tablespoon glycerin

- Mix ingredients together.
- Store in covered jar in the refrigerator for up to 1 week.
- To use, saturate cotton ball and dab on face.

### CREAMY MILK MASK

1 tablespoon buttermilk
1 tablespoon powdered skim milk
4 drops olive oil

- Combine all ingredients.
- Apply to the skin.

- Allow mask to dry and harden for 20 minutes.
- Rinse off with cool water.

### CELL RENEWAL MASK

1 tablespoon yogurt
1 egg yolk
1 teaspoon honey

- Blend all ingredients together.
- Spread on the face.
- Allow mask to dry and harden for 20 minutes.
- Rinse off with cool water.

# FRUIT-ACID PRODUCTS FOR SIMPLE DRY SKIN

**CLEANSERS:**
Pond's Foaming Cleanser
Alpha Hydrox Foaming Cleanser

**TREATMENT PRODUCTS:**
Neutrogena Healthy Skin
Murad Murasome Night Cream
NeoStrata Alpha Skin Smoothing Cream
Formula 405 AHA Facial Day Cream SPF 15
Avon Anew Intensive for the Face
Diane Young Fruit Acid Moisturizer

**TONERS:**
No commercial products formulated for dry skin. Use recipe section at end of chapter to make your own.

**MASKS:**
No commercial products formulated for dry skin. Use recipe at end of chapter to make your own.

## COMPLEX DRY SKIN

All too common in women over thirty-five, complex dry skin is characterized by fine lines, sagging skin, sallow color, enlarged pores, brown spots, and discolorations. The bad news is that these changes are due to a combination of natural aging factors, sun exposure, and cigarette smoking. The good news is that fruit acids can reverse or improve many of the problems of complex dry skin.

Before fruit acids, treatment of complex dry skin consisted of a variety of often expensive, and sometimes painful, techniques to address the different problems—moisturizers to reduce dryness, collagen injections to remove lines, chemical peels to get rid of brown spots, face lifts to improve skin tone, and Retin-A to improve color and flexibility. Properly used, fruit acids can replace many of these techniques, reducing both the expense and side effects such as painful dryness, bright red skin tone, dry eyes, and chapped lips. A combination of home and professional treatments can reduce dryness, restore skin tone, encourage skin growth, shrink pores, diminish fine lines, and return a healthy glow.

|  | FRUIT ACIDS | RETIN-A |
| --- | --- | --- |
| DRYNESS | Improves hydration | Increases dryness |
| DISCOLORATIONS | Gradually fades | Gradually fades |
| SKIN COLOR | Rosy, luminous | Bright red |
| LINES | Decreases fine lines | Decreases fine lines |
| PORES | May decrease size | May decrease size |
| IRRITATION | Slight burning after application | Burning and inflammation |
| SUN EXPOSURE | No problem | Photosensitivity |
| AVAILABILITY | All retail cosmetic outlets and can be made at home | Prescription only |
| ACNE | Opens blocked pores | Decreases oil production; clears blocked pores |

Fruit acids start by removing the top dead layer of skin cells, gradually eliminating dark discolorations and smoothing out skin tone and color. In the dermis, they stimulate the production of new collagen and elastin to restore skin tone and flexibility. Properly used, fruit acids refine and retexturize the skin, producing a luminous quality that you may not have seen since childhood.

To receive the maximum benefits from fruit acids you will need to use the strongest concentration available without a prescription. It might seem odd to use the stronger product for complex dry skin, but it's the right way to go. The multiple problems of dryness, dark spots, fine lines, and enlarged pores require fruit-acid products with enough strength to turn the skin around. This means treatment products that contain between eight and fifteen percent. This might be too strong for some skins, so it can be helpful to start with the lower concentrations and work up to the stronger products.

To begin fruit-acid treatment for complex dry skin you can start with a product like Eucerin Plus, Nivea, or Lacticare, all of which contain around five percent fruit acids. Alpha Ceramide from Elizabeth Arden offers a progressive series of fruit-acid treatments that range from two-and-a-half to five then six percent, preparing the skin for their full-strength seven-and-a-half percent formulation. Once the skin is able to tolerate the lower percentages, you can gradually work up to higher concentration products such as Avon Anew Intensive for the Face (ten percent), Aqua Glycolic (twelve percent), and Murad Murasome Night Cream (eight to fifteen percent).

Milder rinseable cleansers should be used. Two gentle fruit acid–based products are Pond's Foaming Cleanser and Alpha Hydrox Foaming Cleanser. Cleansers without fruit acids that you could use include Neutrogena Cleansing Wash and Oil of Olay Facial Cleanser. Toners are probably not necessary and can be irritating for complex dry skin when using fruit acid products. Fruit acid–based masks can be helpful, but most commercial formulations are designed for oily or normal skin. To fill the need, you can make your own with the recipes at the end of this chapter.

---

## WARNING: FRUIT ACIDS AND THE SUN

Unlike Retin-A, to which they are often com-
pared, fruit acids do not make your skin vulnerable to a bad sunburn. You can use these
products without fear of an angry red burn.
However, the newly revealed skin uncovered
by a fruit-acid peel may be irritated by strong
sunlight. Even if the skin does not indicate sensitivity, it is rather counterproductive to expose treated skin to the sun's rays after you
have worked so hard to clear and freshen your
complexion.

For a safe, even tan use a self-tanner that
contains fruit acids. These products remove the
top dead layer, permitting better penetration
of tanning components.

---

Most dermatologists recommend using a
gentle creamy moisturizer to reduce risk of irritation and excessive flaking. These problems
can happen to any skin type but can be more
common and severe in fine, thin, complex dry
skin. Examples of this type of product include
Eucerin Dry Skin Therapy SPF 25 and Nivea
Visage, both of which offer an extra bonus of
sun protection. At night, soothe the skin with
a gentle moisturizer such as Lubriderm for
sensitive skin, and Moisturel.

## The Next Step

As good as they are, fruit acids have limitations. If you're considering collagen injections or face-lifts, try using fruit acids, both professional and home treatments, for three months. You may see enough improvement to delay the need for additional treatments. If you decide to go ahead with a face-lift your new skin texture will improve surgical results.

## Program of Home Care for Complex Dry Skin

Complex dry skin presents a complex problem. This skin is frequently thin and fragile, but the multiple problems call for a strong fruit-acid treatment program. To deal with both factors, you will need to follow a two-step regimen. In step 1, you will introduce your skin to gentle fruit-acid products that range from three to five percent. If the skin accepts the treatment, you can move up to step 2, stronger six-to-eight-percent fruit-acid creams and lotions. The skin now conditioned by two weeks of gentle fruit-acid treatment will be able to benefit from concentrated treatments without burning and irritation.

## STEP 1: FIRST TWO WEEKS

### NIGHTTIME

1. Remove eye makeup with nonoily cleanser.
2. Wet face with lukewarm water.
3. Squeeze about a half teaspoon of rinseable cleanser into your hand, and work up a lather.
4. Gently massage lather into the skin.
5. Rinse off with 5 handfuls of warm, not hot water.
6. Dry skin gently.
7. Wait 10 minutes.
8. Dot on gentle (3–5%) fruit-acid treatment product.
9. Wait 5 minutes.
10. Smooth on moisturizer.

### Daytime

1. Cleanse with rinseable cleanser.
2. Wait 10 minutes.
3. Apply gentle strength (3–5%) fruit-acid treatment product.
4. Wait 5 minutes.
5. Smooth on moisturizer with sunscreen.

## Step 2

After two weeks of gentle fruit acid therapy—
and if your skin seems to accept the gentle
fruit acid therapy without burning—you can
step up to the stronger 6–10-percent products.

### Weekly Facial

1. Cleanse face with fruit-acid cleanser.
2. Wait 10 minutes.
3. Apply fruit-acid mask for dry skin. Use
   one of the recipes at the end of this
   chapter.
4. Allow mask to remain for 20 minutes.
5. Rinse off with lukewarm water.
6. Splash on a few handfuls of cool water.
7. Wait 5 minutes.
8. Smooth on gentle (3–5%) fruit-acid
   moisturizer.

---

## WARNING: SMOKING AND THE SKIN

Studies have shown that heavy smokers have a paler skin tone and more lines and wrinkles than nonsmokers. Researchers believe that the nicotine in the tobacco slows down blood circulation. This decline means that less food and oxygen are available to the skin cells, while more carbon dioxide is building up in the cells. This unhealthy environment leads to a drastic slowdown in skin growth. Even the best fruit-acid peels and treatment products cannot reverse skin damage if you continue to smoke.

---

## PROFESSIONAL CARE

Complex dry skin can benefit from fruit-acid peels that have been modified to reduce irritation and inflammation. Physicians can change the pH (the acid balance) or even lower the concentrations of the fruit acids in the peel. They may start off with a fifty-percent or even thirty-percent solution that has been adjusted to be less acidic. If the skin tolerates this level, the next step is to gradually increase the treatment time to eight to ten minutes. As the skin becomes stronger, physicians can increase the strength of the peels as well as the length of the time that they remain on the skin. To maintain improvement, they will give their patients home treatment products at varying concentrations, depending on their patients' needs.

---

### ALL SKIN PEELS ARE NOT ALIKE

Don't confuse fruit-acid peels with the far more invasive and sometimes dangerous chemical peels that use phenol or trichloracetic acid. These peels cause burning and crusting that take several weeks to heal. In some cases the peels go too deep and produce scarring. Chemical peels are usually not recommended for dark hair and eyes because these complexion tones tend to develop irregular pigmentation from the procedure. By contrast, fruit-acid peels can be performed on any skin type without scabbing or pain.

---

Recent studies have combined the use of Retin-A with fruit acids. According to Dr. Helen Torok of Ohio, a combination of low concentrations of Retin-A and fruit-acid treatment creams can produce better and quicker results with less irritation than if either product were used alone.

# FRUIT-ACID PRODUCTS FOR COMPLEX DRY SKIN

CLEANSERS:
Pond's Foaming Cleanser
Naturistics Alpha-Natural Skin Renewal
Foaming Cleanser

TREATMENT PRODUCTS—STEP 1 (the first two weeks):
Pond's Age Defying Complex for Delicate Skin
Avon Anew for Chest and Neck
Arden Ceramide 1,2,3

TREATMENT PRODUCTS—STEP 2:
Neutrogena Healthy Skin
Formula 405 AHA Facial Day Cream SPF 15
Murad Night Cream
Aqua Glycolic Face Cream

TONERS:
No commercial products are designed for complex dry skin. Use homemade recipes at end of chapter.

MASKS:
No commercial products are designed for complex dry skin. Use homemade recipes at end of chapter.

## FRUIT-ACID RECIPES FOR COMPLEX DRY SKIN

The recipes for complex dry skin are designed to be gentle and nonirritating, and they can be used as written for both steps 1 and 2. Although there are many excellent commercial fruit-acid treatment lotions and creams, these recipes are the only fruit-acid masks and toner recommended for complex dry skin.

## Complex Dry Skin Shopping List:

Almond oil, aloe gel, apple sauce, beeswax, borax, buttermilk, castor oil, clover honey, coconut oil, egg, grapes, lemon juice, mayonnaise, olive oil, sesame oil, tomato juice, vodka, Vaseline, white wine, white grape juice, yogurt, whole milk.

### BLOODY MARY CLEANSING CREAM

1 teaspoon beeswax
1 tablespoon Vaseline
1 tablespoon castor oil
1 teaspoon coconut oil
1 tablespoon tomato juice
$\frac{1}{4}$ teaspoon borax
1 teaspoon vodka

- Melt wax and oils together in microwave or over low heat if using a stove top.
- Dissolve borax in warm water.
- Beat borax into oil mixture, adding vodka slowly.
- Transfer to small clean jar, and store in refrigerator up to 1 week.
- To use, massage 1 teaspoon into the face.
- Rinse off with warm, then cool water.

### FARMHOUSE CLEANSER

1 egg
1 tablespoon white wine
½ tablespoon olive oil

- Mix egg and wine together.
- Slowly beat in olive oil until mixture is thick and golden.
- Massage into the skin.
- Rinse off with cool water.

### OLD-FASHIONED COLD CREAM

1 tablespoon lanolin
2 tablespoons almond oil
2 teaspoons lemon juice
1 tablespoon aloe gel

- Blend aloe and almond oil.
- Add lanolin and blend over low heat.
- Remove from heat and beat in lemon juice.

- Transfer to clean jar and store in refrigerator.

### CANTON NIGHT CREAM

1 tablespoon liquid lanolin
2 tablespoons sesame oil
2 tablespoons white grape juice
$\frac{1}{4}$ teaspoon borax

- Blend all ingredients.
- Store in small jar in the refrigerator for 1 week.
- To use, massage 1 teaspoon into skin.
- Rinse off with warm water.

### BULGARIAN BEAUTY MASK

$\frac{1}{4}$ cup whole milk yogurt
1 tablespoon clover honey

- Mix together.
- Apply to face.
- Allow to harden for 15 minutes.
- Rinse off with warm, then cool water.

### APPLE MASK

1 tablespoon applesauce
1 egg yolk

- Blend ingredients together.
- Apply to the skin.
- Allow to harden for 20 minutes.
- Rinse off with cool water.

### ARBOR MASK

¼ cup crushed grapes
1 egg yolk
1 teaspoon coconut oil

- Blend all ingredients together.
- Apply to the skin.
- Allow to harden for 20 minutes.
- Rinse off with cool water.

### CELL RENEWAL MASK

1 tablespoon buttermilk
1 egg
½ teaspoon honey
1 teaspoon mayonnaise

- Blend all ingredients together.
- Spread on the skin.
- Allow to remain for 20 minutes.
- Rinse off with cool water.

## MYTH: DIRTY SKIN CAUSES ACNE

The aggressive program long suggested for acne-troubled skin has led to the impression that dirt causes breakouts and if the skin is scrubbed clean acne can be controlled. Not true. It is the oil and cell buildup that clogs and irritates the pores, not soot and grime. In fact, harsh cleansing may actually irritate and provoke more acne problems. A good acne program balances a thorough but gentle cleaning with bacteria controlling agents.

## ACNE-TROUBLED SKIN

Along with college boards, hopeless crushes, and an unlimited craving for pizzas, acne is a seemingly official part of puberty. One of the most frequently encountered skin problems, acne affects up to eighty percent of men and women at some point in their lives. It can consist of blackheads, pimples, enlarged pores, cysts, and in severe cases, scaring.

At the root of the problem are out-of-control oil glands. Difficulties begin when excess oil gets trapped in the follicles and they become inflamed and irritated. In due time, the follicle springs a leak, dumping a mixture of stale oil, bacteria, and blood cells into the lower levels of the skin. If the break occurs near the surface, the blemish is small and short-lived. But if the break is large and deep in the skin, the result is a hard, painful cyst that can lead to a permanent scar.

Traditional approaches attack the problem in a variety of ways. There are soaps that strip off the top layer of dead cells and stale oil that coats the skin. Strong alcohol-based astringents and toners dissolve this oil, while scrubbing grains can slough off skin buildup.

To deal with bacteria that are part of the process, antibiotics are used either orally or topically in oil-free gels and lotions. Salicylic acid, or sulfur compounds are patted on the skin to dry up blackheads and small blemishes. In severe cases of acne, doctors can prescribe Accutane pills or Retin-A gel (both forms of vitamin A acid) to slow down oil gland production. All of these products work well on many people but not without unwanted side effects, and not all the time. The treatments can make the skin extremely dry, sore, and irritated. In some cases, the irritation can provoke breakouts, despite its leaving the skin almost painfully dry.

## INGREDIENTS TO AVOID

Doctors have identified a variety of ingredients frequently used in beauty aids that unsettle oily skin. These include cleansers, moisturizers, hair conditioners, face masks, hand and body lotions, and toners. If you have oily skin, you probably know to avoid creamy, rich products. These are not the *only* substances to avoid. If your skin tends to break out, check the labels of your skin- and hair-care products. Avoiding the substances listed below can go a long way in keeping acne-troubled skin clear and fresh.

Caprylic acid, cetyl acetate, cocoa butter, coconut butter, corn oil, cotton seed oil, glycerol alcohol, hydrogenated vegetable oil, lanolin, laureth-4, lauric acid, myrisstyl alcohol, oleyl alcohol, PEG 16 lanolin, PPG myristyl propionate, propylene glycol, shark liver oil, soybean oil, stearic acid, wheat germ oil.

## FRUIT-ACID HOME CARE FOR ACNE-TROUBLED SKIN

Fruit acids offer a new approach to acne problems. For simple acne that consists of oily skin, blackheads, and small pimples, fruit acids can be used instead of strong soaps and drying lotions. Fruit acids improve the skin by removing the buildup of the excess oil and cells that get caught in the follicles and coat the surface of the skin. Studies have also reported that fruit acids are particularly effective in preventing and reducing the discoloration of healing after acne eruptions.

Cleansers for acne-troubled skin should thoroughly clean the surface of dirt, dead cells, and excess oil, without leaving a residue of oil or wax that can clog pores. The scrubbing grains and sponges that are a time-honored part of acne treatment are too harsh and irritating to the skin when using fruit acids. There are several well-designed cleansers with generous concentrations of fruit acids for acne-troubled skin. Examples of these products include Aqua Glycolic Facial Cleanser and Murad Exfoliant Cleanser. Toners can be helpful to mop up any stray spots of oil and makeup. You can use either fruit acid–based products like Aqua Glycolic Astringent or an alcohol-based formula like Propa-pH or Seba-Nil.

## WARNING: AVOID FRUIT-ACID PRODUCTS THAT CONTAIN WAX OR OILS

The majority of fruit-acid products are designed for dry or older skin. They need the soothing and hydrating properties of a rich, creamy formulation. The acne-controlling properties of fruit acids will be overwhelmed if the product is enriched with oil and/or wax; be careful to select only oil-free fruit-acid products to provide the right environment for fruit acids to work effectively. Don't let anyone talk you into anything else. An overenthusiastic salesperson may try to convince you that the oils in their products will not cause problems. Don't believe it.

The driving force behind any fruit acid based–program is the daily treatment product. This is where and how the skin gets the maximum beneficial effects of fruit acids. Examples for acne-troubled skin include Avon Anew for Problem Skin, M.D. Formulations Glycare, Murad Advanced Oily–Acne Prone Skin, and NeoStrata AHA Solution for oily skin. You may notice an improvement with a few days, but most people say it takes three or four weeks to see the benefits of a fruit-acid acne program. At first you will notice generalized peeling. This is not dry skin but the pores and surface actively shedding the unwanted buildup of cells. When the peeling ends, the skin will look fresher and smoother and existing blemishes will start to disappear. By the end of the month, the skin should be clear of blackheads and the discolorations of old breakouts should be fading rapidly.

## PROFESSIONAL CARE

Fruit acids alone work well for simple acne. For inflammatory acne that includes moderate to large painful red eruptions, fruit acids need to be combined with other methods to bring the acne under control. Physicians usually add antibiotics in the form of lotions or pills, since inflammatory acne always is accompanied by unwelcome bacteria. In other cases, they prescribe Retin-A or Accutane to shut down oil gland production. Doctors find that they can use lower doses of these other treatments (and thus limit unwanted side effects) and still get better results than if either was used alone.

In an office, dermatologists can offer fruit-acid peels to speed up acne control. For home care, they can juggle different treatments depending on the skin's needs. For example, one program can be a combination of office peels and antibiotic lotions, another combination might be a strong fruit-acid cleanser, coupled with antibiotics will both end breakouts and fade scars and discolorations.

## PROGRAM OF HOME CARE FOR ACNE-TROUBLED SKIN

A fruit-acid program for acne-troubled skin may seem almost too simple. There are no hot packs, no facial saunas, no scrubbing grains, and no abrasive sponges. All these steps were used to remove the top layer of dead skin cells. Fruit acids do this without the redness and dryness those time-honored techniques could cause.

### Nighttime

1. If you wear eye makeup gently remove with nonoily cleanser designed for the eye area.
2. Work up a lather with a rinseable cleanser and massage into the skin, wash thoroughly but gently.
3. Rinse face with 10 handfuls of warm water.
4. Dry face gently.

5. Wait 15 minutes.
6. Apply fruit-acid gel.

## Daytime

1. Wet hands and work up lather with rinseable cleanser.
2. Massage gently into skin.
3. Rinse off with 5 handfuls of cool—not cold—water.
4. Dry face thoroughly.
5. Wait 5 minutes.
6. Apply toner with clean cotton ball.
7. Wait 5 minutes.
8. Apply fruit-acid gel.

## Weekly Facial

1. Wash the face with rinseable cleanser.
2. Wait 10 minutes.
3. Apply fruit-acid mask.
4. Allow mask to harden and remain for 20 minutes.
5. Rinse off with cool water.
6. Dry gently.
7. Wait 10 minutes.
8. Apply fruit-acid gel.

After the first few days of treatment you will probably see dry, white flakes on the skin. This does not mean that you have developed dry skin. Rather it is the result of the skin and the follicles actively shedding accumulations of dead unwanted skin cells. When these cells are washed away, the new skin is fresh, clear, and smooth.

## HOMEMADE RECIPES FOR ACNE-TROUBLED SKIN

Fruit acids do not cure acne problems. Instead, they work with other treatments to dramatically improve results. These recipes are to be blended into a program of oil-free soaps, fresheners, and medicated gels.

### Ingredient shopping list:

Apple juice, alum, applesauce (baby), alcohol, buttermilk powder, bran, grapefruit juice, seedless grapes, honey, lemons, rose water, vodka, vitamin C, witch hazel, white wine.

### CITRUS FRESHENER

1 cup boiling water
1 vitamin C tablet
$\frac{1}{2}$ cup rubbing alcohol

- Mix ingredients together.
- Cool to room temperature.
- Store in clean, covered jar in the refrigerator up to 1 week.

### HONEY TONER

1 tablespoon honey
1 teaspoon lemon juice
1 tablespoon rose water
2 tablespoons vodka

- Mix ingredients together.
- Store in clean, covered jar in the refrigerator up to 1 week.

### GRAPEFRUIT FRESHENER

2 tablespoons grapefruit juice
3 tablespoons witch hazel
1 tablespoon alcohol

- Mix ingredients together.
- Store in clean, covered jar in the refrigerator up to 1 week.

## LEMON FRESHENER

2 tablespoons lemon juice
1 tablespoon alcohol
1 tablespoon glycerin
3 tablespoons witch hazel

- Mix ingredients together.
- Store in refrigerator in clean, covered jar up to 1 week.
- To use, saturate cotton ball and apply to skin.

## APPLE ASTRINGENT

$\frac{1}{4}$ cup vodka
$\frac{1}{4}$ cup water
$\frac{1}{4}$ cup apple juice
$\frac{1}{4}$ teaspoon alum

- Combine ingredients together.
- Store in refrigerator.
- Transfer to small, clear glass jar for up to 1 week.

## FRENCH WINE MASK

1 tablespoon white wine
1 egg white
1 teaspoon lemon juice
1 tablespoon buttermilk powder

- Blend everything together.
- Spread on face.
- Allow mask to harden for 20 minutes.
- Rinse off with cool water.
- Wait 10 minutes.
- Apply fruit-acid gel.

## APPLE PIE MASK

2 tablespoons bran
1 tablespoon lemon juice
1 tablespoon baby applesauce

- Combine to make a paste.
- Apply to face and keep mask on for 20 minutes.
- Rinse off with lukewarm water.
- Wait 5 minutes, then apply fruit-acid gel.

## BACCHUS STICKY MASK

$\frac{1}{2}$ cup mashed seedless grapes
1 tablespoon whole wheat flour
1 teaspoon lemon juice

- Mix ingredients together.
- Spread on face.
- Allow to remain for 20 minutes.
- Rinse off with warm, then cool water.
- Wait 10 minutes.
- Apply fruit-acid gel.

## FRUIT-ACID PRODUCTS FOR ACNE-TROUBLED SKIN

CLEANSER:
Freeman's Sugar Cane and Guava Soap
Aqua Glycolic Facial Cleanser
Murad AHA Exfoliant Cleanser

TREATMENT PRODUCTS:
Murad Advanced Oily–Acne Prone Skin
Avon Anew for Problem Skin
M.D. Formulations Glycare 5, 10
NeoStrata AHA Solution for Oily Skin

TONERS:
Aqua Glycolic Astringent
Alpha Hydrox Toner

MASKS:
Freeman's Sugar Cane and Guava Alpha-Hydroxy Peel-Off Mask
Sally Hansen Skin Recovery Purifying Facial Mask
Naturistics Alpha Natural Skin Renewal Facial Mask

# Special Situations

F ruit acids are the chameleons of beauty ingredients. They perform different roles for different problems. Not infrequently, fruit acids work indirectly helping other products do a better job. Researchers have just begun to explore new ways where fruit acids can improve skin and hair quality. This section will explain how and when to turn to fruit acids for help in a wide range of problems.

# BROWN SPOTS AND DISCOLORATIONS

We are all born with clear, smooth, even skin, but after decades of living, this surface shows a variety of brown spots and discolorations. Some, like freckles and liver spots, are the result of unprotected sun exposure. Others, like the brown patches of chloasma, are caused by a combination of medication and sun exposure. Traditional treatments include: burning off individual spots with electric needles, skin peels, and bleaching creams. Raised spots can be removed by scraping with a surgical knife. In recent years, Retin-A creams and gels have helped the skin slough off discolored skin tissue. Unfortunately, Retin-A makes the skin more sensitive to the sun and more likely to develop new discolorations.

Fruit acids have been shown to be particularly effective in many types of discolorations. Physicians apply high concentrations for one or two minutes directly to the spots, and give their patients an eight–twenty-percent fruit-acid cream to use at home. Fruit acids have also been added to prescription lightening creams with excellent results.

Skin lighteners or bleaches don't actually lighten the skin. Instead, they stop the production of melanin, the pigment that causes brown discolorations. As the color fades, the lightening creams prevent new melanin production. Adding fruit acids to skin lighteners helps these formulas do their job more effectively. The fruit acid–enriched lightening creams remove the top layer of dead cells to give the skin-bleaching product better access to discolored areas. In addition, by speeding up cell growth, they help the skin slough off unwanted darkened cells faster. Examples of skin-lightening products that you can order without a prescription are NeoStrata AHA Gel for Age Spots and Murad Advanced Age Spot and Pigment Lightening Gel. Physicians can also ask pharmacists to make up individually designed products that have the same effect as the commercial brands.

### Fruit-acid Skin-lightening Treatment

1. Wash skin with fruit-acid cleanser.
2. Apply lightening gel to dark areas.
3. Allow skin to absorb gel, about 10 minutes.
4. Spread on sunscreen with at least an SPF of 15.

If you can't find a fruit acid–based lightener you can achieve similar results with a two-part program you put together yourself. In the morning apply fruit-acid cream or lotion and a sunscreen. At night use a traditional hydroquinone lightener. Don't combine the two products and use them at the same time. This will cut concentration of each in half, decreasing effectiveness.

---

### FRUIT-ACID PRODUCTS FOR SKIN LIGHTENING

NeoStrata AHA Gel For Age Spots and Skin Lightening
Murad Advanced Age Spot and Pigment Lightening Gel
Lasting Look (distributed by Bio Cosmetic Research Labs)

---

## SENSITIVE SKIN

Is your skin itchy, blotchy, and flaky? Does it tend to develop hives or break out in an itchy red rash? Congratulations, you've got sensitive skin. The sensitivity can be triggered by almost anything in the environment. It can be a problem at any age, for every type of skin. Fine, dry, sensitive skin cannot tolerate traditional cell removal products, like scrubbing grains and Retin-A. Oily, sensitive skins do not react well to drying agents like salicylic acid and alcohol, which are routinely used to control problems of oil production. Skin that is easily irritated may be inflamed by improper use of fruit acids, especially in higher concentrations. To get the benefits of fruit acids without the problems, those with sensitive skin should use extremely mild products with less than five percent fruit acid. You may not see the same degree of quick improvement with the use of these gentle products, but the skin will soften and clear over time.

Alternatively, those with sensitive skin can apply a modified form of fruit acids called Methoxypropylglunamide, mercifully known as MPG. Developed by the Revlon Research

Group, it is found in many of the Time-Off line from Almay and Results skin-care products from Revlon. They have been shown to exfoliate the skin and reduce dryness without irritation. Research is currently underway to learn if this modified form of fruit acid can improve the quality of elastin and collagen in treated skin. They work more slowly, but over time you will be able to see finer texture, line reduction, and smaller pores. The improvement will come slowly, generally over a period of three months of daily use, but without the irritation from traditional fruit-acid products.

## FRUIT-ACID HOME CARE FOR SENSITIVE SKIN

Sensitive skin needs to be introduced gently to fruit acids. Consider your cleansing carefully. Even if your skin tolerated a standard soap, step down to even gentler liquid cleansers when using fruit acids. Good examples of mild cleansers include Cetaphil soapless cleanser, Neutrogena Non-Drying Facial Cleanser, and Aveeno soap for dry or combination skin. Toners, even mild ones, can be irritating when those with sensitive skin use fruit acids. Facial beauty masks can be helpful, but most of the commercial masks may be too strong. Give yourself the benefits of a mask with the following recipes, which are especially mild products that you can make at home.

Fruit-acid treatment products should be used twice a day. If this proves too irritating, start using the fruit-acid product at night for a few weeks, then add a second dose in the morning. Good examples of fruit-acid treatment products for sensitive skin include Almay Time-Off Age Smoothing Moisture Lotion, Avon Anew Perfecting Complex for the Face, and NeoStrata AHA for Sensitive Skin.

When using fruit acids on sensitive skin, you might see a few days of dryness, irritation, and some redness. This reaction means the skin is actively ridding itself of the top layer of dead cells. To relieve dryness and irritation, use a basic moisturizer several times a day. If your skin tends to be oily, use an oil-free moisturizer like Neutrogena Moisture. For dry skin, try nonirritating formulas like Eucerin or Moisturel.

## PROFESSIONAL CARE

Sensitive skin from dry to oily can benefit from fruit-acid peels but the peels must be modified to avoid irritation and burning. Standard peels usually use seventy percent glycolic acid, a concentration that is far too high for sensitive skin. To avoid problems, a physician can dilute the peel to thirty percent and alter the pH to reduce acidity. To decrease chance of irritation, the treatment time is quite short, usually no more than one to two minutes.

Fruit-acid peels can improve the texture of all types of sensitive skin. For dry skin, they can reduce flaking and relieve tightness. Sensitive oily skin, troubled by red, itchy patches and periodic flare-ups, will find fruit-acid peels reduce irritability and breakouts.

# FRUIT-ACID PRODUCTS FOR SENSITIVE SKIN

TREATMENT PRODUCT:
Avon Anew for Chest and Neck
Pond's Age Defying Complex for Delicate Skin
Avon Anew Perfecting Complex for the Face
Almay Time-Off Age Smoothing Moisture Lotion
NeoStrata Sensitive Skin AHA Face Cream SPF 4
Alpha Hydrox for Sensitive Skin

CLEANSERS:
NeoStrata Sensitive Skin AHA Facial Cleanser

TONER:
No product currently available.

MASKS:
No product currently available.

# Men's Skin

At first glance, fruit acids do not hold much of special value for men. Daily shaving ensures excellent cell removal. The skin is naturally thicker and oilier, seemingly more resistant to aging. Even society seems to give men's skin the benefit of the doubt, viewing lines and wrinkles as signs of character rather than aging. Fruit acids, however, do have a place in men's medicine chests.

Their value lies in preparing the skin for a better daily shave. Oil and dirt that accumulate on the skin block the razor's access to the beard. This prevents a smooth shave, which can lead to five-o'clock shadow. For some men, these short, newly-cut hairs grow back around and enter the skin. This appears on the skin as a rash of small red bumps. Removing the top layer of skin cells with fruit acids heals existing problems and prevents their recurrence.

Daily usage of fruit-acid cleansers and lotions prevent buildup of dead skin and increases close contact of the blade during shaving. Without a layer of loose, dead, dry skin, the newly-cut hairs do not become ingrown. If problems do exist, removing this top layer frees the hair and allows the skin to heal.

Men can condition their skin with fruit-acid gels and moisturizers. Younger men should use oil-free products to prevent breakout problems. Men over forty may have drier skin and will benefit from a lotion that improves hydration as well as shaving. Fruit acid–based masks and toners will continue to improve shaving and prevent problems.

As the decades go by, men's skin eventually shows signs of sun damage and aging. Fruit-acid treatments from commercial products, as well as fruit-acid peels from physicians can offer much the same benefits as they do for women's skin. Although daily shaving takes care of cell renewal, fruit acids can improve the quality of collagen, reduce lines, and improve skin tone. There are some excellent products made especially for men. They are often formulated with lower levels of waxes and oils and the fragrances are different than women's products, but the basic action is the same. Men can also use products recom-

mended for women as long as they are formulated for their skin type.

## FRUIT-ACID SKIN CARE FOR MEN

### NIGHTTIME

1. Wash face with fruit-acid soap or cleanser.
2. Wait 10 minutes—watch the end of the
   news or pick out a tie for the morning.
3. Apply fruit-acid gel if face is normal or
   oily, fruit-acid cream/lotion if face is dry.

### Daytime—Electric Razor

1. Apply electric pre-shave conditioner.
2. Shave as usual.
3. Jump into the shower, using fruit-acid
   cleanser or soap on the face and
   deodorant soap on the rest of the body.
4. Towel off and wait 10 minutes. Don't just
   stand there—eat breakfast or get dressed.
5. Apply fruit-acid gel or cream—the choice
   depends on your skin type.

## Daytime—Double-Edge Razor

1. Shower using fruit-acid cleanser or soap on your face, and deodorant soap on the rest of your body.
2. Towel off briskly.
3. Apply shaving gel or cream.
4. Shave as usual.
5. Rinse off and wait 15 minutes.
6. Apply fruit-acid after-shave, gel, or lotion.

# FRUIT-ACID PRODUCTS FOR MEN

**CLEANSERS:**
Pond's Foaming Cleanser
Aqua Glycolic Facial Cleanser
Freeman's Sugar Cane and Guava Soap
Bath and Body Works Renewing Cleanser

**FRUIT ACID–BASED TREATMENT PRODUCTS FOR MEN:**
Aramis Lift-Off Moisturizing Formula SPF 7
Polo Sport Face Fitness AHA
Alpha Hydrox After Shave Lotion for Normal to Dry Skin
Alpha Hydrox After Shave Sensitive Skin Lotion
Avon Anew Performance for Men Complex

**FRUIT-ACID TREATMENT FOR OILY SKIN:**
Pond's Age Defying Complex
Avon Anew Perfecting Lotion for Problem Skin

**FRUIT-ACID TREATMENT FOR NORMAL TO DRY SKIN:**
Lubriderm with alpha hydroxy
Aqua Glycolic Face Cream
Murad Advanced Smoothing Cream SPF 8

# Care of the Body

If you think fruit acids are valuable for the face, wait until you hear what they can do for the body. The thicker skin accepts stronger solutions without the risk of irritation or redness. In addition to banishing dry, itching skin, cracked feet, and flaky legs, fruit acids can improve both hair removal and sunless tanning. In order to appreciate how and why fruit acids work on the body, it is helpful to understand what causes the problems in the first place.

## DRY SKIN 101

At best, we have a very inefficient natural system for moisturizing the skin. The majority of oil glands are in the face and back, and nature's plan is that oil will travel down to the rest of the body. As anyone who has used up jars of body lotion knows, this rarely works. Even women with chronically oily facial skin are bothered by dry, flaky skin on the legs and feet.

The standard approach to the body has been to use bath oils and lotions in what seems to be a losing battle to help skin retain moisture. Body skin, especially on the arms and legs, seems to have an infinite need for hydration. Despite daily applications of rich creams and lotions, dry skin seems to reappear by nightfall. Fruit acids help you get ahead of dry skin. A combination of superfatted soaps, fruit-acid body lotions, and fruit-acid body scrubs and soaps will keep your skin younger and softer.

## WHICH IS BETTER, BATH OR SHOWER?

Bath advocates point to the soothing and relaxing properties of a long quiet soak in the tub. Shower advocates believe that bathing actually can dehydrate the skin and dissolve oils. Truth is, they're both right. A comfortable soak with good bath salts and moisturizers can relieve muscle ache, soothe sunburn, and soften the skin. However if you sit in the bath too long, the skin will become drier. According to Dr. Albert Lefkovits of New York City, a quick shower with lukewarm water will be less dehydrating for older, thinner skin. This is particularly true in low humidity conditions such as cold winter nights or hot, dry sunny days. To bottom line the issue of baths vs. showers, limit soaking time to ten minutes or less in order to get the benefits without the drawbacks.

You do not want to undo the benefits of fruit acids with the wrong cleansers. There are a few fruit acid–enriched body soaps that can be used during both bath and showers. Although these products contain relatively small amounts of fruit acids, they do an excellent job of cleansing the skin and are formulated with an understanding of what fruit acid–treated skin needs. Alternatively, you can use a superfatted soap, like Dove or Basis, so that you will not dehydrate the skin. If you use deodorant soaps, look for those that are enriched with moisturizers to prevent dehydration.

You can make good use of full strength fruit-acid moisturizing formulations for thicker body skin. You should select products that have at least seven to eight percent fruit acids, such as Avon Anew Protecting Complex for the Face and Body, Lubriderm Cream with Alpha Hydroxy Acids, and Vaseline Intensive Care Smooth Legs and Feet. Whatever product you choose to use after bathing or showering, dry off and wait ten minutes before applying the fruit-acid moisturizer.

## FRUIT-ACID TREATMENT FOR THE BODY

### Basic Care:

1. Clean body with fruit-acid soap.
2. Dry thoroughly.
3. Wait 10 minutes.
4. Apply fruit-acid cream or lotion.

## Intensive Weekly Treatment:

1. Wash body with fruit-acid soap.
2. Massage a homemade body scrub into skin, paying close attention to the knees, elbows, and feet.
3. Rinse off thoroughly.
4. Dry briskly with thick terrycloth towel.
5. Wait for 10 minutes.
6. Apply fruit-acid cream or lotion.
7. If skin tends to be rather dry, smooth on a gentle moisturizer as well.

## HAIR REMOVAL

Fruit acids act in an indirect way when waxing or shaving. The top dead layers of skin cells tend to interfere with hair removal. These cells block access to the base of the hair, so by removing this layer prior to hair removal, you will produce a smoother and longer-lasting shave. Similarly, fruit acid–treated skin allows leg wax to have better contact with the root of the hair and remove the hair more easily with less pain.

To improve hair removal, use a fruit-acid lotion prior to shaving or waxing. After the procedure, however, it is better to wait twenty-four hours before using a fruit-acid product again to prevent irritation. Instead, use a mild moisturizer, such as Moisturel or Lubriderm (for sensitive skin) after waxing or shaving.

## SUNLESS TANNING

Fruit acids have been shown to promote quicker, deeper sunless tans because treated skin can absorb more tanning chemicals faster and more evenly. The top dead layer of skin cells create a lumpy barrier to the self-tanning creams. The result? The skin absorbs the tanning chemical unevenly, creating areas of light and dark pigments. Because the tanning cream sits on this dead surface it is more likely to wear off more rapidly.

If you use fruit acids regularly, continue to use your favorite self-tanning product. If you use a traditional body lotion, there are self-tanners that contain fruit acids. Estée Lauder has introduced two products, Self-Action Super Tan and Origin Summer Vacation that, according to the company, cut the time of tanning in half.

## WARNING: PROTECT DELICATE SKIN FROM FRUIT ACIDS

Recent news reports have cautioned that fruit acids can irritate vaginal or rectal tissues. To avoid problems, do not use fruit-acid cleansers in these areas. In the tub or shower use a traditional bath bar for sensitive areas, and the fruit-acid soap or cleanser on the other areas such as arms, legs, and face.

## FRUIT-ACID RECIPES FOR THE BODY

The thicker, drier skin on your legs and body responds beautifully to the fruit acids. The scrubs and smoothers combine a bit of abrasion with the fruit acids to remove dry, flaky skin on feet, legs, and elbows. The milk-based bath soaks (these contain lactic acid) gently loosen dead, dry skin on the arms, back, and chest. The herbal conditioner and sparkling cleanser are refreshing ways to smooth and refresh the skin. Try the milk baths in cold, windy weather and the cleanser when you're hot and sticky.

## Ingredient Shopping List for the Body:

Yogurt, wheat germ, coconut oil, honey, buttermilk, peach kernel oil, club soda, lemon juice, cinnamon, cloves (ground), apple juice, whole milk yogurt, clay, whole wheat flour, rosemary (dried), thyme (dried), mint (dried), apple cider vinegar, fennel, oat bran (ground), millet flour, grapes.


### YOGURT BODY SCRUB

2 cups yogurt
1 tablespoon wheat germ
1 tablespoon coconut oil
1 tablespoon honey

- Blend ingredients together.
- Rub all over the body, leave on for 5 minutes.
- Shower off thoroughly with warm water.


### MILK BATH

2 cups buttermilk
1 tablespoon peach kernel oil

- Blend ingredients together.
- Add mixture to warm bath.
- Soak for 20 minutes.
- Rinse off in cool shower.

### SPARKLING CLEANSER

2 cups club soda
2 tablespoons fresh lemon juice

- Combine all ingredients.
- Gently sponge on body, leave on for 5 minutes.
- Rinse off with lukewarm water.

### SPICY MILK BATH

2 cups buttermilk
2 tablespoons honey
$\frac{1}{2}$ teaspoon cinnamon
$\frac{1}{2}$ teaspoon ground cloves

- Blend ingredients together.
- Add mixture to a warm bath.
- Soak for 20 minutes.
- Dampen washcloth in the tub and rub over the skin.
- Stand up, drain tub, and rinse off with cool water.

### MOISTURIZING BODY SCRUB

4 tablespoons lemon juice
4 tablespoons apple juice
4 tablespoons yogurt
1 tablespoon clay

2 tablespoons wheat germ
2 tablespoons whole wheat flour

* Blend first four ingredients.
* Add rest of ingredients; stir until ingredients are combined.
* Standing in a tub, massage mixture all over the body; leave on for five minutes.
* Rinse off in lukewarm shower.

### CLEOPATRA MILK BATH

2 cups boiling water
1 tablespoon dried rosemary
1 tablespoon dried thyme
1 tablespoon dried mint
1 cup whole milk yogurt

* Add herbs to boiling water.
* Steep for 30 minutes—strain, saving liquid.
* Combine liquid (it's called an infusion) with yogurt.
* Stir into a warm bath.
* Soak in bath for 20 minutes.
* Rinse off under shower.

### VINEGAR HERBAL BODY CONDITIONER

1 cup water
$\frac{1}{2}$ teaspoon dried rosemary
$\frac{1}{2}$ teaspoon dried thyme
$\frac{1}{2}$ teaspoon dried mint

½ teaspoon dried fennel
1 cup apple cider vinegar

- Combine water and herbs and bring to a boil.
- Add vinegar and let herbs steep for 24 hours.
- Pour ½ cup into a shallow bowl.
- Dampen sponge with vinegar infusion and dab on legs and arms, with special attention to knees and elbows.
- Rinse off in a lukewarm, then cool, shower.

### ORGANIC BODY SMOOTHER

1 tablespoon ground oat bran
2 tablespoons millet flour
1 tablespoon wheat germ
1 cup mashed grapes
1 teaspoon peach kernel oil
Lemon juice as needed

- Blend oat bran, millet flour, and wheat germ with oil.
- Dilute with lemon juice to make a paste.
- Rub on knees and elbows.
- Rinse off with cool water.

# FRUIT-ACID PRODUCTS FOR THE LEGS AND BODY

TREATMENT PRODUCTS:

Avon Anew Perfecting Complex for Face and Body
Freeman's Sugar Cane and Guava Lotion
Lubriderm Cream
Aqua Glycolic Hand and Body
NeoStrata AHA Skin Smoothing Lotion
Lacticare
M.D. Formulations Night Cream
Murad Advanced Skin Smoothing Lotion
Lac-Hydrin Five
Vaseline Intensive Care for Smooth Legs and Feet
Alpha Hydrox Lotion
Formula 405 AHA Moisturizing Body Lotion, SPF 15

CLEANERS:

Alpha Hydrox Body Wash for Dry Skin
Alpha Hydrox Body Wash for Normal Skin
Naturistics Alpha Natural Facial Soap
Freeman's Sugar Cane and Guava Soap

## THE HANDS

We subject our hands to constant abuse. They are dunked in soap suds, dried out with dust and paper, seared by the sun, and buried in garden dirt. Hands don't take this treatment quietly. They rebel with dryness, chapping, redness, brown spots, and roughness. Most of these problems are the result of a lack of moisture. Standard cures have been to drench the hands in round after round of creams and lotions—still it can seem like a losing battle. Less than thirty minutes after massaging in cream, hands can feel tight and rough again.

Fruit acids will revolutionize the way you care for your hands. Once a day treatment with fruit acid–enriched cream or lotion will repair even chronically dried and reddened hands. Fruit acids remove the dry, chapped cells while helping the skin to build up moisture. Unlike traditional products that rely on oils to form a film on the surface, fruit acids stimulate the production of natural moisturizing factors (NMFs) to hold water throughout the skin in the hand. Even when challenged by harsh soaps and drying dust, fruit acids help the skin hang on to necessary moisture.

There are over a dozen effective fruit-acid hand and body creams currently available. Excellent examples include Lubriderm AHA, Vaseline Intensive Care Lotion for Smooth Hands and Feet, and Avon Anew for the Body. For best results, use the cream after washing the hands. The residual moisture in the hands will be retained by the fruit acids and the creams. Normally, you would need to wait ten to fifteen minutes between washing your skin and applying fruit acids in order to avoid irritation. In this case, the thicker skin on the hands is less susceptible to irritation and can tolerate fruit acids on freshly washed skin. If your hands are especially dry, apply a fruit-acid cream at night, pull on a pair of beauty gloves, and go to sleep. In the morning, the hands will have a softness that lasts for days.

When you have the time, use a homemade hand soak for long-lasting softness and freshness. Use the recipes at the end of this chapter.

## Fruit-acid Treatment for Dry Hands

1. Wash hands with fruit-acid soap.
2. Apply hand care mask (see recipe section).
3. Rinse off thoroughly with cool water.
4. Dry gently.
5. Wait five minutes.
6. Apply fruit-acid hand cream.

## Fruit-acid Treatment for Age Spots

1. In the morning, massage fruit-acid cream into the hands.
2. At night, following manufacturers instructions, apply skin-lightener to the top of the hands.

### FRUIT-ACID RECIPES FOR THE HANDS

Cooking up hand-care recipes at home will not just save you money—it will create extraordinary hand masks and soaks unavailable in any drug or department store.

## Ingredient Shopping List:

Applesauce, borax, Crisco, egg yolk, glycerin, grapes, liquid lanolin, lemon juice, olive oil, peach kernel oil, tomato juice, Vaseline, white wine, yogurt.

#### BEECHNUT HAND CREAM

3 tablespoons Crisco
1 tablespoon baby applesauce
½ teaspoon borax

- Melt Crisco over low heat.
- Beat applesauce into Crisco until creamy.
- Dissolve borax into applesauce in a separate pot.
- Store in a clean, covered jar in the refrigerator for up to 1 week.

### NEAPOLITAN HAND CREAM

2 tablespoons Vaseline
1 tablespoon tomato sauce
$\frac{1}{2}$ teaspoon borax
1 teaspoon glycerin

- Melt Vaseline over low heat.
- Dissolve borax into tomato sauce in a separate pot.
- Stir in the glycerin.
- Beat tomato sauce mixture into Vaseline until creamy.
- Transfer to clean jar and store up to 1 week in refrigerator.
- To use massage one teaspoon into hands.

### LEMON AID FOR ELBOWS

2 tablespoons lemon juice
2 tablespoons glycerin
$\frac{1}{2}$ teaspoon borax

- Blend ingredients together.
- Apply to the elbows.

- Leave mixture on overnight. To protect your sheets wear a long-sleeved nightgown.

### EGG CREAM FOR ELBOWS

1 egg yolk
1 tablespoon white wine
½ tablespoon liquid lanolin

- Blend ingredients together.
- Massage into elbows.
- Wrap elbows with plastic wrap.
- Leave on for 20–40 minutes, depending on your schedule.
- Wipe off residue to avoid staining clothes.

### GRAPE HAND SOAK

3 tablespoons yogurt
¼ cup seedless grapes, crushed
1 teaspoon glycerin
1 teaspoon peach kernel oil

- Blend ingredients together.
- Pour into a shallow bowl.
- Soak hands in the mixture for 20 minutes.
- Every few minutes, massage the mixture into the hands and cuticles.
- Wash off with superfatted soap.
- Dry hands.

## NAPA VALLEY HAND MASK

1 egg, beaten
1 tablespoon white wine
1 teaspoon olive oil

- Blend all ingredients together.
- Massage into hands.
- Cover each hand with a small plastic bag.
- Keep bags on hands for 1 hour.
- Wash hands with superfatted soap.
- Dry hands.

## THE NAILS

The nails are made of keratin, the same hard protein found in skin and hair. Nails that lack water become brittle and fragile. They tend to peel, chip, and break easily. Not infrequently, household cleaning products or overuse of nail polish solvents can dry out and make the nails fragile. As the years go by, the nails become increasingly brittle, part of the increasing dryness that is experienced throughout the body.

Traditional care has focused on the use of hand creams and lotions to hydrate the nails. During a routine manicure, the nails are massaged with cream. Unfortunately, since nails must be free of any oil before applying polish, the hand cream must be removed completely with a strong solvent, like acetone, before continuing the manicure, and thus undoing the value of the cream. Once the polish is in place, it is difficult for creams to affect or even reach the actual nail.

Fruit acids can help both the nails and the cuticles. They can remove dead, dry nail cells that shorten the life of the manicure. These cells tend to flake off, taking layers of polish

with them. In addition, fruit acids can increase
nail strength by encouraging water retention.
If your nails break and peel easily, fruit-acid
treatments can make them strong and long.

In addition to improving the health and
strength of the nails, fruit acids can shape and
control the cuticle. Although cuticles interfere
with the perfect manicure, they protect the nail
bed from infections. Aggressive cleaning with
instruments can expose the nail to bacteria
and other organisms. For this reason, most
doctors caution against cutting the cuticle during a manicure. Fruit acid–enriched products
safely dissolve the excessive dry cuticle without exposing the nail to unwanted organisms.
During a manicure, you can use fruit acid–enriched creams, such as Sally Hansen AHA Cuticle Remover, Avon Advanced Miracuticle,
and Cutex Manicare, or you can use one of the
recipes that follow. You will be amazed how
well you can control the shape of your cuticles
without cutting.

## FRUIT-ACID CARE FOR THE NAILS

To receive fruit-acid benefits, the nail must
be free of polish. If you always wear polish,
your best choice would be to use fruit acid–
enriched cream during a manicure. To improve results, massage the cream into the nails

and wait for fifteen minutes before continuing the procedure. If you plan ahead, take off your polish the night before a manicure. Massage a generous amount of fruit-acid cream into the nails, cover with a beauty glove, and go to sleep. The next day, your nails will be well hydrated, stronger, smoother, and better able to hold onto your polish.

If you go for months between manicures, fruit acids can keep your nails strong and healthy without regular attention. You can use fruit-acid hand and body lotions or make your own hand treatments and soaks to improve nail quality. Retail products, including Lacticare, Lubriderm, and Vaseline Intensive Care, will deliver first quality fruit-acid benefits. If you have a few extra minutes, warm up the lotion for great penetration. Brittle or peeling nails respond well to intensive fruit-acid treatments. Soaking nails in these formulations will strengthen and smooth even chronically fragile nails.

Traditional nail hardeners frequently contain formaldehyde. While these products can be effective, they can cause problems. In some cases, formaldehyde has been shown to provoke severe reactions, such as nail discolorations and bleeding in the nail bed. Fruit acids do not create problems, and they impart strength to the nails.

## The Fruit-Acid Manicure

1. Shape nails with emery board.
2. Soak fingers in a cuticle reducing solution (see recipe section).
3. Rinse in lukewarm water.
4. Slightly warm fruit-acid cream (you can use commercial or homemade formulation).
5. Massage warm cream into hands.
6. Cover hands with small plastic bags, secure.
7. Keep bags on for twenty minutes.
8. Wash hands with fruit-acid soap.
9. Apply base coat and polish as usual.

## FRUIT-ACID RECIPES FOR THE NAILS

There is simply nothing on the market like the fruit-acid products you can make at home for the nails. These easy-to-make formulas will change the way you care for your nails. They will eliminate the need for cutting the cuticles and help the manicure to last longer.

## Ingredient Shopping List for Nails:

Buttermilk, baby applesauce, borax, canned crushed tomatoes, egg yolk, olive oil, oatmeal

(ground), peach kernel oil, spirits of peppermint, safflower oil, wheat germ, white wine,
yogurt (whole milk).

### ROMAN NAIL SOAK

$\frac{1}{2}$ cup crushed tomatoes
1 teaspoon olive oil
2 teaspoons white wine

- Combine all ingredients.
- Pour mixture into cake pan.
- Dip nails into mixture.
- Soak for 20 minutes.
- Rinse off, rubbing cuticles with dry
  washcloth.

### BULGARIAN CUTICLE SOFTENER

3 tablespoons whole milk yogurt
1 teaspoon safflower oil
1 drop spirits of peppermint

- Combine all ingredients.
- Rub into cuticles.
- Rest hands on a clean towel for 20
  minutes.
- Wash off with superfatted soap, rubbing
  cuticles with dry washcloth.

## BUTTERMILK NAIL RUB

2 tablespoons buttermilk
2 teaspoons wheat germ
2 tablespoons bran

- Combine all ingredients.
- Massage gently into cuticles, and leave on for 5 minutes.
- Rinse off with warm water.
- Rub cuticles with thin cotton dish towel.

## APPLE NAIL MASQUE

2 tablespoons baby applesauce
1 tablespoon rice flour
1 teaspoon peach kernel oil

- Combine all ingredients.
- Massage into nails.
- Cover hands with small plastic bags.
- Leave bags on for 20–25 minutes.
- Rinse off with warm water while rubbing nails with nail brush.
- Wash with superfatted soap.

## LOIRE VALLEY CUTICLE CREAM

3 tablespoons white wine
1 egg yolk
1 teaspoon olive oil

- Beat ingredients together.
- Massage into cuticles.
- Pull on cotton beauty gloves and go to sleep.
- In the morning, scrub nails gently with nail brush.
- Rinse off. Wash with fruit-acid soap.
- Massage in fruit-acid hand cream.

### OVERNIGHT LEMON TREATMENT

Juice of one lemon
1 tablespoon powdered oatmeal
1 teaspoon peach kernel oil

- Combine all ingredients.
- Spread on cuticles.
- Pull on cotton beauty gloves.
- Leave on gloves for at least six hours or overnight.
- In the morning, rinse off with superfatted soap and warm water.

## FRUIT-ACID PRODUCTS FOR THE NAILS

Sally Hansen AHA Gel Cuticle Remover
Avon Advanced Miracuticle Vanishing Complex
M.D. Formulations for Nail and Cuticle
Cutex Manicare
Pfizer Manimagic

## THE FEET

We ignore our feet. We pull on socks, stick our feet into shoes, and hope for the best. While most women will diligently cleanse and moisturize their face and body, very few people spend even a tenth as much time caring for their feet. Make no mistake about it, the feet don't take kindly to this lack of attention. They rebel with constant dryness of the skin around the ankles, and thick, hard calluses on the soles of the feet. Dryness on the upper part of the foot is a result of lack of oil glands, a problem for all the extremities. Without a layer of oil, the feet cannot maintain a healthy supply of water in the skin. Socks are part of the problem because they absorb moisture. They're designed to do that. But when they strip away moisture from the surface of the skin, it promotes dryness. If you walk around your house barefoot or wearing sandals, the dust or dirt on the floor actually acts like absorbent powder, drying out the feet even more.

## MYTH: HIGH-HEELED SHOES CAUSE FOOT CALLUSES

Narrow, tight, and arched shoes with high, thin heels are frequently blamed for the development of thick, hard calluses on the soles of feet. These shoes may be uncomfortable and definitely are not made for walking, but the truth is calluses can come from the majority of shoes. Even traditional comfort shoes like loafers, clogs, and molded sandals will not protect the foot from the pounding of routine walking. The one shoe that offers protection? It's the heavily cushioned running shoe with two or three inches of flexible padding and support. This is not a shoe to wear with an Italian suit or a silk dress, but it works well if you're on your feet for hours.

Hard, dry calluses on the bottom of the feet occur when natural dryness combines with body stress. The callus is a protective response to the pounding that the feet receive from daily walking. The cells build up to protect the bones and the more delicate structures of the foot.

People often blame shoes for this callus buildup, but shoes have been excessively maligned. In fact, there are few shoes that will not promote the development of calluses. Even special sandals, which are designed for better balance and less pressure when walking, can promote callus development because they expose the foot to more dirt and dust.

Traditional care of the feet has focused on the use of moisturizers for the top and bottom of the foot and scraping with pumice stones and razor blades to remove the calluses. Podiatrists can also prescribe orthotics, specialized shoes or shoe inserts. These devices redistribute body weight to make walking less irritating to the soles of the feet. Podiatrists caution against scraping away calluses with a knife or razor. This so-called bathroom surgery can produce dangerous infections.

Fruit acids and the feet are made for each other. The hard, dry skin responds beautifully to the highest strengths of alpha hydroxy acids. Not only do they encourage the skin to hold water by increasing the natural moisturizing factors, but they are perfect for removing the calluses safely without any risk of irritation or inflammation. Without cutting or scraping, fruit acids dissolve a callus enough so that it can be rubbed off with simple and safe pumice stones.

For best results, choose hand and body lotions that contain at least eight percent fruit acids, such as Alpha Hydrox for the Body, Vaseline Intensive Care for Smooth Hands and

Feet, and Avon Anew for the Body. Problem Feet by Freeman is a fruit-acid scrub that does an excellent job of both removing dead cells and improving hydration.

Fruit acids work well, but they are not instant cures. The feet must be treated repeatedly with fruit acids for about a week to soften a callus before its removal, but it is remarkable how much smoother and softer the skin will be after a fruit-acid and pumice treatment. If you apply your fruit acids at night and top them with clean cotton socks, the fruit acids will do their job quicker and more efficiently.

## PROGRAM OF FRUIT-ACID CARE FOR THE FEET

### Nighttime

1. Wash feet with superfatted soap like Dove or Basis. Don't use a deodorant soap, which can be too dehydrating.
2. Dry feet thoroughly.
3. Massage in 1 tablespoon of fruit-acid cream or lotion per foot. Rub it into both the top of the foot as well as the soles.
4. For best absorption, pull on clean thin cotton socks.
5. Go to sleep.

## Daytime

1. After morning bath or shower, apply 1 teaspoon of fruit-acid cream to your feet.
2. Every five days, use a pumice stone or scrubbing grains on the soles.
3. Work a nail brush over the toenails to groom excessive cuticles and dead skin.
4. Rinse off thoroughly.
5. Dry well, using a rough towel to pick up loose skin.
6. Wait 5 minutes.
7. Apply an additional dose of fruit-acid cream or lotion.

## Fruit-Acid Treatment Soak

If you jog or are simply on your feet a lot, try a weekly soak to soften and refresh your feet.

1. Wash feet with superfatted soap.
2. Pour a foot soak (see recipe section) into dishpan.
3. Submerge feet.
4. Relax. Watch TV or read the paper for 30 minutes.
5. Every few minutes, massage a bit of the mixture into the foot.
6. After 30 minutes, rinse off.

7. Dry thoroughly with thick terry towel.
8. Massage 1 tablespoon fruit acid into each foot.
9. Pull on a pair of clean thin cotton socks.
10. Go to sleep.

## FRUIT-ACID RECIPES FOR THE FEET

Until now there hasn't been too much that we could do for dry, hard, calloused feet. Creams and lotions hardly made a difference. Professional pedicures sliced and slashed at hardened skin, that grew back all too quickly. Until you've tried a fruit-acid foot soak or scrub, it will be hard to believe how well they work. The skin will feel softer almost immediately. After several days treatment, the dead hard skin is easily rubbed off with scrubbing grains and pumice stone.

## Ingredient Shopping List for the Feet:

Almond oil, alum, apple juice, beeswax, buttermilk, castor oil, cocoa butter, eggs, glycerin, lemons, liquid facial cleanser, mint leaves (fresh), parsley (fresh), peach kernel oil, red wine vinegar, rosemary, sunflower oil, safflower oil, vodka, white wine, yogurt (whole milk).

## HERBAL FOOT BATH

$\frac{1}{2}$ cup water
$\frac{1}{2}$ tablespoon fresh rosemary leaves
$\frac{1}{2}$ tablespoon parsley leaves
Juice of one lemon
3 cups water

- Boil $\frac{1}{2}$ cup water, add herbs.
- Allow herbs to soak for 2 hours.
- Strain, reserving liquid.
- Combine herb infusion and lemon juice.
- Combine with 3 cups of water.
- Pour into dishpan.
- Immerse feet in tub, rubbing with washcloth.
- Soak for 20 minutes.

## INVIGORATING FOOT RUB

2 tablespoons sunflower oil
4 tablespoons red wine vinegar
$\frac{1}{2}$ teaspoon alum powder
2 drops camphor oil

- Combine all ingredients.
- Massage into the feet.
- Rest feet on a clean towel.
- After 30 minutes, wash off with warm water.

### DRY FEET CARE CREAM

1 tablespoon glycerin
2 tablespoons lemon juice
2 tablespoons apple juice
1 teaspoon castor oil

- Combine all ingredients.
- Massage into feet.
- Slip on a pair of cotton socks.
- Go to sleep, or go to work.

### WILLIE WONKA FOOT RUB

4 tablespoons cocoa butter
1 ounce beeswax
4 tablespoons almond oil
2 tablespoons white wine

- Melt all ingredients together in a microwave.
- Beat until creamy.
- Pour into clean glass jar, store in refrigerator for up to 2 weeks.
- To use, rub 2 teaspoons into feet.
- Pull on a pair of clean socks and go to sleep.

## RUSSIAN FOOT SOAK

1 cup yogurt (whole milk)
2 tablespoons vodka
1 cup water

- Combine all ingredients.
- Soak feet for 30 minutes.
- Wash off with superfatted soap.
- Smooth on fruit-acid lotion.

---

### FRUIT-ACID PRODUCTS FOR THE FEET

Freeman Barefoot
Vaseline Intensive Care for Smooth Legs and Feet
M.D. Formulations Pedicare Cream
Avon Anew for the Body
Alpha Hydrox for the Body

# THE HAIR

The hair is made of the same keratin protein as skin and nails so it's not surprising that fruit acids can be of help to a range of hair and scalp problems. The surface of the hair shaft is made up of a series of overlapping scales, much like the shingles on a roof. When the hair is soft and shiny, the scales lie flat and smooth. If the hair is dry and brittle, the scales are raised and jumbled. Hair naturally has a flat, smooth surface, but after frequent bouts of blow-drying, straightening, coloring, and perming, the surface becomes raised and ruffled.

Traditional hair treatments use protein shampoos and rich conditioners to coat the hair shaft and flatten the bumpy surface. The traditional treatment certainly works to a point, but fruit acids can improve the performance of these products. In many cases, the dead, dry cells of the hair stand up and are raised and ruffled. Conditioners just press them down, leaving the hair shaft still bumpy, uneven, and looking and feeling stiff. Fruit acid–enriched shampoos remove the dead cells and actually clean up the hair surface.

Fruit-acid conditioners work particularly well with hair that tends to be oily. Rich protein shampoos can leave oily hair limp and stringy even a few hours after washing, leading to extra cycles of washing, blow-drying, and damage. Fruit acids will remove the buildup on the hair shaft, but do it without oils that flatten your hair.

On the scalp, fruit acids are reported to offer additional benefits in dandruff control. Ideally, the scalp cells pass through the stages of growth in an orderly fashion. When they reach the scalp surface, they are dry, dead, and ready to fall off. Regular brushing and washing will remove these cells, and dandruff flakes will not appear. When this orderly pattern is not followed, too many cells arrive together at the surface. Too numerous and too tightly packed together, they cannot be dispersed by regular care. The result: The cells stick together and fall out in clumps that we call dandruff.

Standard antidandruff shampoos use keratolytic agents designed to dissolve dead cells. These can work well, but not for everyone. Many women do not like the way these shampoos smell or the way they leave the hair. For women who have lightened, straightened, or permed hair, many antidandruff shampoos can be far too strong and damaging. For others the shampoos simply don't work, and the scalp remains dry and flaky.

Fruit acids, as they do in so many other situations, take an alternative approach. Shampooed into the hair and scalp, they dissolve the glue that holds the cells together, permitting them to be rinsed away. But the fruit acids don't stop there. They help the scalp produce natural moisturizing factors to rehydrate the area, preventing cells from drying out prematurely.

Fruit-acid treatments for the hair are hardly new. Lemon juice has been used for centuries to condition and shine the hair. Despite the inherent value to the scalp, there are relatively few commercial hair-care products with fruit acids. These include Aqua Glycolic Cleanser by Herald, Pure Elements Balancing Shampoo, and Lissée Natural Essence of Orange Organic Shampoo. These products should be massaged into the scalp and then rinsed off.

Fruit-acid hand and body lotions can be adapted into excellent conditioners for dry and color-treated hair. Fortunately, fruit-acid conditioners, rinses, and treatments for all types are among the easiest and most effective products you can make at home.

## Program of Fruit-acid Care for the Hair

1. Wash hair with shampoo designed for your hair type.
2. Towel dry.
3. Apply a treatment pack (or look to recipes that follow).
4. Be sure to massage the pack into the scalp.
5. Allow the treatment to remain for 20 minutes.
6. Rinse out thoroughly with shampoo designed for your hair type.

## FRUIT-ACID RECIPES FOR THE HAIR

These recipes provide a unique opportunity to create products that are not available in a store. Despite the benefits of fruit acid there are few if any products for the hair and scalp. Fruit acid–based conditioners are terrific for oily hair, while hair masks can restore shine and flexibility to dry hair. The dandruff treatments can be adjusted for different hair needs.

## Ingredient Shopping List for The Hair:

Apple cider vinegar, chamomile (dried), egg, lemon juice, mineral water, olive oil, rice vinegar, rosemary (dried), sage (dried), tomato juice, witch hazel.

### GIBSON GIRL HAIR RINSE

1 cup apple cider vinegar
1 cup mineral water

* Combine all ingredients.
* Pour over freshly washed hair.
* Massage into hair and scalp, and leave in for 5 minutes.
* Rinse out thoroughly.

### HERBAL HAIR RINSE

1 cup water
1 cup rice vinegar
1 teaspoon dried rosemary
1 teaspoon dried camomile
1 teaspoon dried sage
2 tablespoons lemon juice

* Boil water.
* Add herbs.
* Steep for 1 hour.
* Strain, reserving liquid.
* Combine with vinegar.
* Pour over freshly washed hair.

- Massage into the scalp, leave in for 5 minutes.
- Rinse out thoroughly.

### DRY SCALP DANDRUFF TREATMENT

1 tablespoon vinegar
1 tablespoon warm water
1 tablespoon olive oil (for dry hair)

- Combine all the ingredients.
- Massage into scalp.
- Allow mixture to remain for 10 minutes.
- Wash with rich shampoo, rinse thoroughly.

### SUNSHINE HAIR RINSE (FOR OILY HAIR)

Juice of one lemon
Juice of one lime
1 tablespoon witch hazel

- Combine all ingredients.
- Pour over freshly washed hair.
- Massage into the scalp.
- Keep mixture on for 15 minutes.
- Rinse thoroughly.

### ROMANY TREATMENT MASK (FOR OILY HAIR)

1 cup tomato juice
1 egg white

- Whip ingredients together until foamy.
- With a fresh, one-inch paint brush, apply mixture to the hair.
- Keep mixture on the hair for 20 minutes.
- Wash out thoroughly.

### TUSCAN TOMATO MASK (FOR DRY HAIR)

1 cup of tomato juice
1 egg yolk
1 teaspoon olive oil

- Whip ingredients together.
- Dab mixture on the hair with a small natural sponge or cotton ball.
- Keep on for 20 minutes.
- Wash hair with moisturizing shampoo, then rinse thoroughly.

# FRUIT ACID PRODUCTS FOR THE HAIR

SHAMPOO:

Pure Elements Balancing Shampoo for Normal or Oily Hair

Freeman Alpha Enzyme Treatment Shampoo (controls dandruff)

Pure Elements Hydrating Shampoo for Dry or Treated Hair

Lisee Natural Essence of Orange Organic Shampoo

CONDITIONER:

Lisee Essence of Orange Organic Conditioner

Pure Elements Hydrating Conditioner

Pure Elements Daily Detangler

# THE EYES

The eyes are the most delicate and sensitive part of the body. To prevent damage, we have developed a series of protective devices. To shield the eye from danger, the skin around the eye is loose, soft, and thin, able to close up quickly to shield the eye from irritants. Exposure to smoke, strong sunlight, and irritating fumes trigger the skin around the eye to snap shut. While this protects vision, the constant motion of this loose skin contributes to early wrinkling and aging around the eyes. Under the eye, the thin, flexible skin tends to fill up with fluid in response to allergies and irritations. For sun protection, the under-eye skin has the ability to produce melanin, a pigment that darkens the skin to shield it against the sun's rays. This darkening contributes to the dark shadows under the eyes.

## WARNING: PROTECT THE EYE AREA FROM SUN DAMAGE

It is hard to overestimate the damage that the sun can do to the skin around the eyes. It loosens the skin over and under the eyes, etches lines at the corners, and produces dark shadows under eyes. Doctors recommend making an eye-area sunscreen a regular part of the daily wake-up routine. After washing your face and brushing your teeth, pat on a light layer of sunscreen. You can add additional protection with sunscreen-enriched makeup, including foundation, eye shadow, and concealer. When you plan to stay out in strong sun, slip on a pair of shades to broaden protection. Remember, if you don't protect your eyes from the sun, the best fruit-acid products in the world can't keep up with the constant damage from new sun exposure.

Traditional care for the eyes recognizes the unique characteristics of the thin skin around this area. Many products that can be used successfully on other parts of the body cannot be applied in the eye area. Moisturizers can be a particular problem because when they bring water to the skin, they can actually increase puffiness above and under the eyes. Many of the most successful eye-care products are in a sense astringents that actually decrease the puffiness and clarify the skin around the eye. Sunscreens are equally valuable in eye-care products because they diminish the melanin production under the eye, as well as protect the eye skin from the aging rays of the sun.

The eye area can really benefit from the toning and firming qualities of fruit acids, but the skin is too delicate to accept the stronger formulations. Consequently, most body and facial fruit-acid products cannot be used around the eyes. There are a handful of products that have been modified to improve the eye area without provoking problems. Some, like Anew Perfect Eye Care offered by Avon, use a lower percentage of fruit acids. You will not see the quick improvements that you get with stronger products on other parts of the skin, but over time there will still be noticeable benefits. Other products, like Almay Time-Off Age Smoothing Eye Cream and Revlon Results Brighten-Up Eye Cream use a modified form of fruit acid designed to both stimulate cell renewal and reduce dryness without stinging or irritating. This form of fruit acids is also used in products developed for sensitive skin. Another approach, such as that used by Murad, uses a full strength formulation of fruit acids, but reduces the acidity to decrease chance of inflammation.

The limited number of fruit-acid eye-care products might tempt you to try one of the milder face and body lotions for this area. Don't do it. The eyes are especially vulnerable to infection and can become red and inflamed easily from contaminated beauty aids. Even the low levels of bacteria that build up in cosmetics and will not affect the rest of the body will irritate the eyes.

---

## MYTH: FACIAL EXERCISE CAN REDUCE LINES AND WRINKLES AROUND THE EYES

This is a tough one. No one disputes that exercise can build up and tone muscles on the legs, arms, and torso. On the face it's another story. The exaggerated facial expressions like puffing out the cheeks or arching the eyebrows do not give the facial muscles the same kind of workout that weight-bearing exercise produces for the rest of the body. In fact, these so-called facial exercises actually increase wear and tear on facial collagen or elastin fibers and can actually accelerate wrinkling and sagging.

---

To avoid these problems, cosmetic executives have wisely marketed eye-care items (including those with fruit acids) in small containers that often have tiny openings. The small-sized package, usually less than two ounces, is designed to be used up quickly, before bacteria can grow to dangerous levels. The small opening allows you to squeeze out what you need without touching the product with your fingers and contaminating it with dirty hands.

Fruit acid–enriched eye-care products can be used in the morning, after you cleanse your face, and/or at night before you go to sleep. As with all eye-care products, it is wise to date them and discard after three months. Try to remember to wash your hands before using these products so that you do not bring bacteria into the jar or rub it in the eye area. If irritation does develop in this area, you may be particularly sensitive to fruit acids and should discontinue using the product for the eye area. This certainly does not mean that you have to discontinue using fruit acids for the rest of the body.

There are no fruit-acid recipes included at the end of this chapter because of concern for contamination, safety, and irritation. Products designed for the eye area are best developed under sanitary manufacturing conditions that comply with public health manufacturing codes.

## FRUIT-ACID PRODUCTS FOR THE EYES

Avon Anew Perfect Eye Care Cream
NeoStrata Sensitive Skin AHA Eye Cream
Almay Time-Off Age Smoothing Eye Cream
Murad Murasome Eye Complex
Revlon Results Brighten-Up Eye Cream

# Questions and Answers

**Q. Are fruit acids safe to use every day?**
A. Fruit acids have been used for over twenty years in different product formulations. There is no evidence to indicate they cause unwanted side effects or long-term problems. Unlike many new products that come out, fruit acids actually have a long history of experience. Although the way we are using them today is slightly different and at somewhat higher concentrations, doctors believe that we have enough experience with fruit acids to provide a feeling of security in their use.

**Q. I have thin, sensitive skin. Can I use fruit acids?**
A. Sensitive skin requires modified forms of fruit-acid products. You need either to have very gentle concentrations (two to four per-

cent), or you need to use a modified form of fruit acids. Alternatively, some products reduce the acidity of the fruit-acid products to make them less irritating to sensitive skin. You have to be your own judge. If you start off using very mild, gentle products and you don't have problems, you can continue to use them. But if your skin becomes irritated, inflamed, splotchy, or you feel a burning sensation that lasts for more than a moment, then you're going to have to look for other ways of treating and caring for your skin.

**Q. Can I use a hand-and-body fruit-acid product on my face?**
A. Fruit-acid products for the hand and body are frequently strong, with higher concentrations of the fruit acids or more acidity than facial products. Because the skin on the body and on the hands is thicker and tougher, it can handle these stronger formulas that range from eight to twelve percent. If you do not have sensitive skin you can use a hand-and-body product successfully on your face. One final thought: These products may contain higher levels of oils and wax than a product designed for the face. Facial creams and lotions are designed to be worn under makeup. Using a hand-and-body formulation on your face might turn powder or foundation orange

and streaky. If they are used at night, this will not be an issue to worry about.

## Q. Do I need a moisturizer if I use a fruit-acid product?

A. That's an interesting question. Fruit acids are superb moisturizers so it seems odd that most cosmetic companies either include moisturizing agents in the product or encourage the use of a second moisturizer. But moisturizers do have a real place in fruit-acid treatment. These products are a source of moisture for the fruit acids to hold on to. If there is no moisture in the skin, then the fruit acids can't hydrate the skin. Additionally, they reduce chances of irritation from the fruit-acid products, encouraging fruit acids to do their job without discomfort. If you have oily skin, be careful to use oil-free moisturizers to avoid provoking blackheads and breakouts.

## Q. How much should I pay for a fruit-acid product?

A. The value of a fruit-acid product depends not on its price but on its concentration and formulation. There are many excellent products that are less than two dollars an ounce. There are also good products that are forty dollars an ounce. I personally don't feel comfortable using a product that is twenty times the cost of an equivalently effective one. My suggestion would be to look for the least expensive product that gives you the results you want.

## Q. Can I use fruit acids around my eyes?

A. Yes, but use only fruit-acid products designed specifically for the eye area. Unfortunately, there are a very limited number of them. Remember the eye's skin is one of the most sensitive parts of the body, and that you need to use either a very either low concentration or a low acidity in the formula. In addition, you need to take into consideration the special preservative needs of eye-care products. Eye-care products need to have low levels of preservatives—so that they won't be irritating—and are sold in small, hard-to-contaminate packages. Be very careful in choosing such products for the eyes. If you experience discomfort, return the product to the manufacturer.

## Q. What soap should I use when using fruit acids?

A. The choice of soap depends on your skin type. But as a rule, you should step down the type of cleansing you're using when you add fruit acids to your beauty routine. For example, if you have normal skin and you use traditional bar soap, you probably want to switch to a liquid cleanser for normal skin that is less irritating and less dehydrating. If you have oily skin, you may well be using a strong degreasing soap and/or cleansing grains. Abrasive cleaners were very important in the care of oily skin before we had fruit acids, but few skins can tolerate strong scrubbing products in addition to using fruit acids. It is best to step down to a milder cleanser for oily skin. If you have dry skin and use bar soap (even a superfatted one) you will probably need to switch to a rich, creamy water soluble cleanser.

**Q. I'm confused. What's the difference between low acidity and percentage of fruit acid in a product?**
A. It is confusing. Fruit-acid products work best in an acidic environment. Unfortunately, acids can be very irritating and hard to tolerate for most types of skin. Cosmetic chemists need to adjust the acidity to balance the effectiveness of the fruit acid while keeping the base of the product comfortable to use.

**Q. Can I use a toner when I use fruit acids?**
A. It depends on your skin type. Oily skins can use a toner while normal skins may find it's not necessary. With any other skin type it is probably be best to start off without using a toner, then see how the skin looks and feels.

And if there is still an unwanted level of oiliness, you can add a mild toner.

**Q. How can fruit acids help both oily and dry skin?**
A. Good question. And the answer is that fruit acids actually normalize the skin. For oily skin, the fruit acids remove the top dead layer of skin cells, allowing the oil to flow out of the follicle where it can be easily removed without stripping the skin of healthy cells and essential moisture. In the case of dry skin, the fruit acids remove the dead, dry skin that piles up on the surface. This stimulates cell renewal, encouraging the growth of young, healthy cells.

**Q. My skin is oilier in the summer and drier in the winter—should I change the type of fruit acids I use?**
A. Definitely. You need to be sensitive to the effect of weather changes on your skin. In the summer, you may want to add a toner to your fruit acid–based treatment. In the winter, you might want to switch to a milder cleanser. Be aware that the quality of your skin varies from season to season, day to day. You should adjust your skin-care routine accordingly.

**Q. Can I use fruit acids in the sun?**
A. Fruit acids don't cause the same kind of photosensitivity reaction (that angry redness)

one develops from Retin-A, but this isn't an invitation to bake yourself. Be aware that because the fruit acids remove the top layer of skin and are themselves sometimes irritating, they can leave your skin more vulnerable to sun damage. People should always use sunscreens when exposed to the sun's rays, and fruit acid use is just another reason to protect your skin. There are actually several fruit-acid products that also contain sunscreen, such as Formula 405 AHA Moisturizing Body Lotion SPF 15.

**Q. How can fruit acids help the hair? Won't they dissolve it?**
A. There has not been as much research on their effects on hair so far, as there has been with the skin. Preliminary studies have shown that fruit acids remove both the dandruff scales that build up on the scalp and the dead, dry cells that coat the hair's surface. Fruit acids dissolve the glue that holds dead, dry cells together and not the cells themselves. This is much less damaging than keratolytic agents like sulphur or salicylic acid that are frequently the active ingredients in dandruff shampoos.

**Q. Can hands use a stronger fruit-acid treatment than the face?**
A. Yes, because the hands have a thicker and

tougher skin, they can use a higher concentration without inflammation. Most hand creams contain between eight and fifteen percent fruit acids.

**Q. How do fruit acids differ from enzymes that break down the dry skin?**
A. Enzymes like bromelain, papain (from papayas), or salicylic acids are beta hydroxy agents that act by dissolving the dead, dry cells. By contrast alpha hydroxy acids dissolve the glue that holds dead cells together, increase hydration of the skin, and encourage the repair of elastin and collagen. While the fruit enzymes have been shown to dissolve the dead, dry layers that stimulate cell renewal, they have not been shown to increase hydration or improve collagen and elastin.

**Q. How often should I use fruit acids if I'm trying to lighten my skin?**
A. You can use fruit-acid lighteners twice a day.

**Q. I have diabetes. Can I use fruit acids, or will the irritation be dangerous for me to use on my feet and hands?**
A. There is no evidence that fruit acids can be a problem for diabetic skin. In fact, they can be beneficial in relieving the thickening dry skin that builds up on the hands and the soles of

the feet. A moderate strength (five to eight percent) fruit-acid cream, can do an excellent job of softening chronically-rough, dehydrated skin.

**Q. Can people of color use fruit acids?**
A. You are wise to be concerned. The full-strength seventy-percent-fruit-acid peels have been shown to produce discolorations in people of color. To avoid these problems, Dr. Cherie Detrie of Philadelphia suggests starting with a twenty-percent peel, gradually raising the concentration if all goes well. Commercial products usually contain five to twelve percent fruit acids and should not produce discolorations at these strengths. To be safe, start off with the mildest products and work your way up to the stronger formulations. If you develop any irritation, stop use immediately. If you have particularly sensitive skin and are prone to develop dark spots, try a fruit-acid product first in an inconspicuous area such as inside your arm or thigh.

**Q. Can I use fruit acids if I'm pregnant?**
A. There is no evidence to indicate that fruit acids are dangerous during pregnancy. But some doctors, like Dr. Albert Lefkovits of New York, who has extensive experience with fruit acids, do not feel comfortable recommending fruit acids during pregnancy. It's more of an

example of what we don't know at this point
than what we do know, and it is better to err
on the side of safety. Dr. Lefkovits points to
the fact that salicylic acid which is a keratolytic agent, and used to dissolve dead, dry
cells, is related to salicylic acid or aspirin,
which has been shown to cause problems during pregnancy. To be on the safe side, it is better to avoid fruit acids (like almost any other
medications) during pregnancy.

**Q. How often should I get fruit-acid peels?**
A. Physicians usually recommend a four- to
eight-week series of fruit-acid peels, followed
by booster peels every three months. This will
remove the top, dead layer, increasing hydration, improve tone and texture without taking
too much time or money.

**Q. Can I shave my legs after I use fruit-acid
peels?**
A. Yes. Fruit acids improve the shave because
they allow the razor better access to the hair
shaft. Immediately after shaving, it is best to
use a mild non–fruit acid product to avoid irritation.

**Q. Who should get a fruit and skin peel?**
A. Professional peels provide benefits for a
wide variety of skin problems. It can reduce
fine lines and wrinkles, create a more lumi-

nous tone. improve texture, diminish pores, discourage breakouts, and relieve dryness. The peel must be adjusted by an experienced dermatologist to deliver benefits and avoid problems.